Managing a Dental Practice

THE GENGHIS KHAN WAY

Second Edition

Managing a Dental Practice

THE GENGHIS KHAN WAY

Second Edition

Michael R. Young, BA BDS MSc

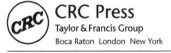

CRC Press
Taylor & Francis Group
Boca Raton London New York

CRC Press is an imprint of the
Taylor & Francis Group, an **informa** business

CRC Press
Taylor & Francis Group
6000 Broken Sound Parkway NW, Suite 300
Boca Raton, FL 33487-2742

CRC Press is an imprint of Taylor & Francis Group, an Informa business

No claim to original U.S. Government works

International Standard Book Number-13: 978-1-910227-66-4 (Paperback)

This book contains information obtained from authentic and highly regarded sources. While all reasonable efforts have been made to publish reliable data and information, neither the author[s] nor the publisher can accept any legal responsibility or liability for any errors or omissions that may be made. The publishers wish to make clear that any views or opinions expressed in this book by individual editors, authors or contributors are personal to them and do not necessarily reflect the views/opinions of the publishers. The information or guidance contained in this book is intended for use by medical, scientific or health-care professionals and is provided strictly as a supplement to the medical or other professional's own judgement, their knowledge of the patient's medical history, relevant manufacturer's instructions and the appropriate best practice guidelines. Because of the rapid advances in medical science, any information or advice on dosages, procedures or diagnoses should be independently verified. The reader is strongly urged to consult the relevant national drug formulary and the drug companies' and device or material manufacturers' printed instructions, and their websites, before administering or utilizing any of the drugs, devices or materials mentioned in this book. This book does not indicate whether a particular treatment is appropriate or suitable for a particular individual. Ultimately it is the sole responsibility of the medical professional to make his or her own professional judgements, so as to advise and treat patients appropriately. The authors and publishers have also attempted to trace the copyright holders of all material reproduced in this publication and apologize to copyright holders if permission to publish in this form has not been obtained. If any copyright material has not been acknowledged please write and let us know so we may rectify in any future reprint.

Library of Congress Cataloging-in-Publication Data

Names: Young, Michael R. (Michael Robert), 1953- , author.
Title: Managing a dental practice the Genghis Khan way / Michael R. Young.
Description: Second edition. | Boca Raton : CRC Press/Taylor & Francis, 2016.
| Includes index.
Identifiers: LCCN 2016003386 | ISBN 9781910227664 (alk. paper)
Subjects: | MESH: Practice Management, Dental
Classification: LCC RK58 | NLM WU 77 | DDC 617.60068--dc23
LC record available at http://lccn.loc.gov/2016003386

Visit the Taylor & Francis Web site at
http://www.taylorandfrancis.com

and the CRC Press Web site at
http://www.crcpress.com

Printed and bound by CPI Group (UK) Ltd, Croydon, CR0 4YY

Contents

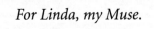

For Linda, my Muse.

Foreword

I would recommend this book to everyone working in dental practice, and more importantly tell them to keep it handy as it is a great revision tool. Little gems of advice pop out at you just when you need them and the book also has the ability to make you think beyond the obvious and to consider other items and issues you could work on to improve your business.

I found the second edition of *Managing a Dental Practice the Genghis Khan Way* a great revision tool and an aid to my own development and understanding of the complexities of managing a practice in the 21st century. The book has been a pleasure to read and along the way it has helped me update my own management skills, before then putting Mike's useful tips to work in my own practice.

This book is a well put together step-by-step guide for all levels of manager. For the more competent or experienced manager it is a reference tool, a checklist against which to benchmark your own personal development plan, as well as being a superb aide-mémoire. The busy manager will have no difficulty finding exactly what they want as the book is very reader-friendly, and every topic is presented in a straightforward manner that is so easy to find.

As a new manager or leader the book will be very easy to read and understand. There are step-by-step action plans for you to follow, with great advice on what to do and what *not* to do, as well as highlighting some of the pitfalls.

This brilliant book is comprehensive and covers all aspects of management that you could possibly need in your day-to-day role. It also helps you see, experience and learn from just about every situation you might come across in your practice.

The book has reminded me how important it is to review your actions, and that we all need to constantly learn and improve within our job if we are going to help our business grow and develop.

It is great that Mike has 'learned the hard way' on our behalf and been able to share his experience and knowledge with us. Thank you Mike for the advice you have offered in this wonderful book.

Niki Boersma
President
Association of Dental Administrators and Managers (ADAM)
October 2015

Preface

This book is for anyone who either owns or aspires to own a practice, and for everyone involved in managing a dental practice. Its aim is to show you how to turn your practice into a successful business. It is a 'How to . . .' book for survival in the business of dentistry. Among other things it will show you the importance of teamwork and communication, of staying close to your patients, keeping ahead of the pack, and of continuous prudent financial management.

I have not set out to show you how much I know, but rather to make you think more about what you are doing, and perhaps help you come up with innovative ways of doing things that are more suited to your circumstances. The book is intended to provide you with a toolkit of concepts, ideas and methods relevant to understanding how to successfully manage a dental practice. It will develop your knowledge and hopefully act as a springboard for further exploration and study of the all-pervading world of management.

No two practices are ever the same: they are infinitely variable and invariably complex organisations in which people interact, and in which the simultaneous processes of delivering dental care and managing a business coexist. The best anyone writing about managing such a complex organisation can hope for is that they make the reader think, and this is why I have scattered a number of 'Hold this thought' suggestions throughout the text, which are all designed to make you think that little bit harder about what you have just read. In some places, some of the topics are only discussed in outline; this is deliberate because they are meant to stimulate your thinking, hopefully in a new direction.

What are the differences between this edition and the one published in 2010? All of the original book has been revised and updated. There is a new section on buying and setting up a practice, as well as much more about managing patients and employees. Included in managing employees you will find information about leadership, working with other clinicians, and more about team building. I have in places rearranged some material, and overall I have expanded parts of the book.

You will not be surprised to know that the section on policies and procedures now includes a chapter on how to manage the Care Quality Commission, a body that had only just come into existence at the time I was writing the first edition, but which is now a very big and very important part of practice management. I thought it unnecessary to include yet another lengthy text on what the Care Quality Commission does or with what dental practices have to comply. I have therefore kept this side of the discussion to a minimum and have instead focused on *how* practices can comply, which seemed to me to be more important than *why*.

All in all, I believe the second edition is a much broader and more up-to-date version of the first.

The book is set out in five main sections: Preparation; Purchase; People; Planning; Policies and Procedures. I have retained 'A final thought'.

The parallel aims of a dental practice are the delivery of excellent patient care (which can only be delivered if you have well-trained and highly motivated employees) and the maximisation of income and profit. Sound management of all of the resources of the practice is essential. Unfortunately, very few practice owners take the time to step back and analyse what is really happening to their business. The day-to-day short-term problems of running the practice almost inevitably take priority over medium- and longer-term business planning.

Why *Genghis Khan*? Well, Genghis Khan was the leader of the Mongols in the late twelfth and early thirteenth centuries. His military strategies included gathering good intelligence and understanding the motivation of his rivals. He was quick to learn and to adopt new technologies and ideas. Legend has it that he was always to the forefront in battle. His ambition was to expand the Mongol Empire and to conquer the world. He united people: he improved communication within his empire through the introduction of a single writing system and, by bringing the Silk Route under the control of one political system, he helped foster communication between Asian and European cultures. Although the West thinks of him in negative terms, he is one of history's more charismatic and dynamic leaders.

Whichever way you look at it, you will need all of Genghis Khan's tenacity if you are going to make a success of being a dentist *and* a business owner.

Managing a dental practice, or when it comes to it, any business, is not about being a dictator: you sometimes have to be gentle, while at other times you will have to be severe and firm. You have to run your practice like an iron fist inside a velvet glove. This is why my advice might at times seem contradictory, in one place suggesting that you have to be ruthless, and at other times telling you to be more empathetic. As in life, business is never black and white; there are always grey areas.

Making a success of managing a dental practice demands clear vision, broad business knowledge and an understanding of a rapidly changing world. It also requires a mastery of your tools and techniques. Above all, it demands wise judgement.

I make no apologies for mentioning some things more than once: this is because first they are important; and, second, because no part of managing a practice exists in isolation. I have continued to present some of the information as bullet points, because according to the proverb, 'One word is enough for a wise man.'

I have had to present some information, such as legislation, regulations and processes, as it is at the time of writing, but I have tried to keep this to a minimum because no matter how things might change, the underlying principles of practice management will I believe always remain the same. I hope this book will teach you those principles so that no matter what problems you may face in the future, you will hopefully be able to find a solution. Why not aim to be an excellent manager as well as an excellent dentist?

I have continued to include many of my own experiences (good and bad), and some of those of my friends and former colleagues, which I hope adds a realistic feel to the narrative. My anecdotes, which are written in a more conversational style, are displayed in boxes. In many ways this book reflects my own odyssey through the choppy waters of practice ownership.

This should not be the only management book you ever read. Although I hope my book becomes your main source of inspiration, there are many more books from which you can extract additional knowledge. As in the practice of dentistry, you should never stop searching for new and better ways to manage your practice.

Michael R. Young
October 2015

About this book

The purpose of this book is to provide a framework, advice, help and guidance for anyone who is now, or is likely to be at sometime in the future, either directly or indirectly (at whatever level) responsible for managing a dental practice. The groups of readers it is therefore aimed at are as follows:

- The dental student who is about to qualify.
- The newly qualified dentist.
- The associate working in practice.
- The associate who is thinking about buying or setting up their own practice.
- The single-handed practitioner or partnership who is looking for ways to improve the management of their practice.
- The larger practice that is looking for ways to improve the management of the practice.
- The Dental Bodies Corporate (DBC) that wants ways to improve the management of individual practices within the organisation, or of improving the management of all of their practices right across the board.
- Dental Care Professionals (DCPs).
- Practice managers, both those who have full management responsibility and those who perhaps feel they want to be able to contribute more.
- Dental receptionists who have aspirations to one day manage a dental practice.
- Dental nurses who have aspirations to one day manage a dental practice.
- Any non-dental managers who are interested in moving into dental practice management.

Basically, this book contains something for everyone working in a dental practice, no matter what stage of their career he or she is at.

The book is intended to provide information about how to manage every type of dental practice.

- NHS
- private
- a mixture of NHS and private
- single practice
- multiple (group) practices
- general
- single specialist
- multiple specialist
- single-handed and partnerships
- multiple-handed
- owner-managed
- company-owned and managed.

This was never intended to be a theoretical management book; it is a warts-and-all guide to managing a dental practice, written by someone who has been there, made mistakes and survived. I hope the reader can learn from my experiences.

I couldn't make up my mind whether to refer to the people you treat as patients or customers; in places it seemed more appropriate to call them patients and in others to call them customers. In the end I decided to call them both, depending on the context. I also couldn't decide whether to refer to the people who work in a practice as employees, staff, or team. Again, I use all three depending on the context.

Acknowledgements

This book might have my name on the cover, but I could not have written it without the help and support of a number of people, all of whom have generously given me their time and have freely shared their thoughts.

Steve Campbell, of Nexus Dental Laboratory, helped clarify my ideas about working with dental technicians. Helen Targar RDH and Heather Lonergan RDH both shared their thoughts about the working life of a dental hygienist. Susie Anderson-Sharkey of Dental FX, a practice manager, enlightened me about the day-to-day challenges she faces in her role. Dr Carol Sommerville Roberts BDS MFDS of Evolve Dental, who gave me greater insight into the challenges facing practices when it comes to complying with the Care Quality Commission. A big thank you also goes to Dr James Robson BDS of Identity Individual Dental Care, for allowing me to spend time at his practice and for letting me take up so much of his practice manager's time.

Two people who deserve a special mention are Ann Gilbert Dip. Dent. Hyg. and Stacey Firman, who shared both their time and their knowledge with me about the workings of the Care Quality Commission. Ann's in-depth understanding of the principles of CQC was invaluable, as was Stacey's grasp of the day-to-day workings of and problems associated with CQC in a practice setting.

A number of other people and organisations provided me with information about, among other things, the practice buying process, the role of the specialist accountant and the specialist dental solicitor, project management, and of course the role of the practice manager. My thanks go to Alan Suggett, Amanda Maskery, Sandra Tavares, Derek Watson, Caroline Holland, Steve Lavelle, Debbie Edwards, Lauren Rosenstone, Natasha Oxley, Andy Jakeman, Malcolm Swan, and the Association of Dental Administrators and Managers.

Once again my wife, Linda, took on the job of proofreading and of generally tidying up the manuscript before I submitted it to the publisher. Along the way we had many lively discussions about what I should say and how I should say it, but the end result was always better with her input than it would have been without. Thank you, Linda.

Finally, I would like to thank everyone at Radcliffe Publishing for having sufficient faith in me to commission a second edition, and everyone at CRC Press who were ultimately responsible for its publication.

Remember, to be successful you don't have to be perfect;
you just have to be better than the rest.

Section I

Preparation

What is practice management?

Before anything else, preparation is the key to success.

(Alexander Graham Bell)

Management is simply the action of managing. It is a noun, but the verb 'manage' (and its derivatives 'manages', 'managing' and 'managed') means:

- to be in charge of people or an organisation
- to succeed in doing something
- able to cope despite difficulties
- to control the use of money and other resources.

The best working definition of management I have come across is that it is 'Getting things done through other people'.

You can see that as the owner and/or manager of a dental practice you will need to be able to do all of the above: be a great leader; be successful despite the occasional (or perhaps frequent) difficulties; and an accomplished controller. However, perhaps most importantly, if you want people to do what you want them to do *and* do it well, you are going to have to be an excellent communicator.

Hold this thought: at the heart of every excellently managed business is excellent communication.

However, management is not just about telling people what to do and/or how to do it: that might work in the short term, but if you are going to build a long-term business you also need to build a long-term team.

Hold this thought: the foundation of a successful practice is a great team.

Management is not a black art, but like all disciplines it has its own language. Once you understand the language then the fundamentals of management are very simple.

There are basically four simple stages or steps in any management process.

- Planning: first, you decide on a particular course of action to achieve a desired result.
- Organising: next, you gather together all of the resources that will be needed to achieve the result.
- Implementing: you then get other people to work together smoothly and to the best of their ability as part of a team to do the work.
- Controlling: finally, you monitor, review or measure the progress of the work in relation to the plan and take steps to correct things if they are off course.

This is no different to the process you go through tens of times a day when you treat your patients.

Planning is perhaps the most important stage, because if your planning is not right, everything else that follows will also not be right.

Hold this thought: the management of anything follows the 'Planning, Organising, Implementing, Controlling' cycle.

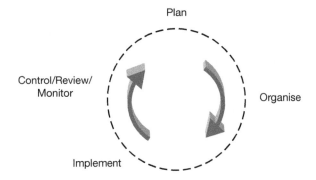

Figure 1.1 The management cycle

In reality, you will find yourself moving from planning to organising, but then going back and tweaking your plan, and doing the same when you eventually move on to implementing. It is a continuous circle of fine tuning.

Learn to be a manager

Perhaps just as important as acquiring your practice is knowing what to do with it once you have ownership. Your practice is not going to manage itself, nor are the staff going to recruit and train themselves. You should therefore have the necessary management and leadership skills *before* you became a practice owner, not after.

How many young (and some maybe not-so-young) dentists become practice owners having had little, if any, management experience? You wouldn't dream of practising dentistry without having first been fully trained, so why become a manager without first gaining the necessary knowledge and experience?

You should by now have found an excellent accountant and an excellent solicitor to give you financial and legal support. The final piece of the jigsaw is managerial support: it's now time for you to start acquiring management skills and knowledge, and an understanding of what is going to be involved in running your own business.

There are literally thousands of books about management, ranging from 'The simple guide to . . .' to heavier academic tomes on management theory. Find a fairly straightforward, well-written (which will make it easier to understand) book and read it. There are also numerous books on 'How to start your own business'. Buy one of these and read it. You should always be prepared to read new things and always be looking to increase your understanding of management and business.

After you have gained some basic knowledge of management, you might want to try some management courses, both generic and ones specific to dental practice. Courses give you the opportunity to ask questions and to mix with and talk to other like-minded people. The best part of some courses is not always what you learn in the formal teaching sessions, but what you find out during informal conversations with other delegates during the coffee and lunch breaks.

Hold this thought: you will have a better chance of succeeding as a practice owner if you find out beforehand what running a business is all about, rather than leaving it until after.

What do you need to know about? In a very broad sense, you'll need to know about:

- the practice of management
- dental practice management
- how to manage people
- how to manage all kinds of resources
- how to manage money.

Many people fail to manage (or manage to fail!) because whenever they are trying to accomplish anything they go straight to the implementation stage, leaving out planning and organisation. They usually compound the problem by also failing to control or review the process on an ongoing basis. The result is that the outcome is not what was hoped for. A great deal of time, energy and money is therefore wasted, and people's frustration levels rise.

Managing a dental practice is really no different to managing any other professional business. You need to think of practice management as being made up of two essential and inevitably linked processes.

- Management of the patients.
- Management of the business.

By the time you are considering setting up on your own you should have mastered how to manage patients, whether it be a single-visit, simple course of treatment, or a complex, multi-visit course of treatment. However, not only must you be a competent clinician, but you must also know how to manage your business.

Management of the business involves knowing how to manage:

- employees, which includes associates, hygienists and therapists, treatment coordinators (TCO), receptionists, and the people doing your lab work, the dental technicians; don't forget that you might have to also manage a manager
- resources of all kinds, and knowing how to maximise their use
- finances, and working within your budget.

It also involves knowing how to plan for the short, medium and long term.

There are your employees who must be managed, from recruitment to departure. On the positive side this will include their training and development, objective setting and performance reviews (appraisals). On the negative side it might involve disciplinary action or dismissal.

Money has to be managed so that the practice makes a profit and so it can pay its bills. This means that you have to set budgets, prepare cash-flow forecasts, and know how to avert financial disaster.

The premises you work in need to be managed so that they are safe and welcoming. This means having a rolling maintenance programme, not just for the building, but also for the fixtures and fittings.

There are also outsiders to be managed: technicians, suppliers, specialists (practice and hospital-based), employment and recruitment agencies. Learning how to work with these people so that your practice gains maximum benefit from their products and skills is critical.

Lastly, but perhaps most importantly, you should learn how to manage yourself.

You might ask, 'Why should I bother to manage my practice?' The simple answer is, 'A well-managed practice is not only nicer to work in, but in the long term it will probably be more successful. It will also certainly be less stressful!'

The way you manage your practice is very much up to you. However, the style I advocate throughout this book is one of teamwork, which to some of you may go against the grain ('It's my practice and I'll run – or is that ruin – it how I want!' I can hear you say). Your way may work in the short term, but if you want a practice that is going to be successful in the longer term, teamwork is going to be the only way to do it.

Hold this thought: dentistry is all about teamwork.

I didn't bother to find anything out about management until I'd been a practice owner for about 10 years, but once I realised its importance I devoured book after book on the subject. I wasn't so much interested in the latest management theory or reading the words of the latest management guru. What I wanted to learn were the underlying principles, the how and why.

Once you have made the decision that you really want to run your own practice give yourself a 'gap' (Get All Prepared) year in which to lay the foundations for your new venture, *then* start looking for somewhere to buy or to set up in.

Not wanting to start out on too much of a negative note, but here are some of the commonest mistakes people will make when they set up a new practice:

- failing to thoroughly research the market beforehand. The current owner may have survived quite happily where they are for years, but if there's another recently opened practice in the area, are you going to enjoy the same easy ride?
- not having a high-quality business plan, which contains marketing and financial plans. Successful businesses all start out with a detailed, carefully worked out business plan
- not listening to professional advisers. You're paying them for their expertise, so listen to what they have to say
- setting their sights too high in terms of location, size of premises, or quality and quantity of fixtures and fittings
- over-investing in fixed assets. Don't sink all of your money into capital equipment; keep cash back to cover running costs and to ease your cash flow
- failing to employ the right people
- not learning how to be a manager beforehand.

Hold this thought: failure to research and plan does not necessarily mean your practice will fail; it might, however, mean that it takes longer to be a success.

Section II

Purchase

2

Do you really want to own a practice?

Buy in haste, repent at leisure.

(Adapted from a proverb, 1693)

Not every dentist wants to work in a practice let alone own one, but if your ambition is to be your own boss you need to have some idea of what you are letting yourself in for. Buying or setting up a practice is a major personal, professional and serious financial commitment. The purpose of this chapter is to make you stop and think before you take this giant step.

The first thing I want to do is set out some of the thoughts that lie behind the purchase or setting up of a practice, the starting points from which you can navigate your personal pathway through what can be a minefield. I say 'you' because no two people's experiences can ever be the same, although there will of course be common threads and similarities. This section will throw lots of questions at you and hopefully provide some answers.

- Why do you want to own a practice?
- Who should *not* own a practice?
- When is the best time to buy a practice?
- Where's the best place to look for a practice to buy?
- What sort of practice will you be looking for?
- How is the price of a practice determined?
- Where's the best place to look for finance?
- What's the best way of securing finance?
- Do you know how to write a business plan?
- What are the common problems with business plans?
- What's involved in the process of buying a practice and what can go wrong?
- Who else will you have to involve?
- How do I go about refurbishing the practice?
- Do I need to incorporate my new practice?
- Where is the best place to set up a new practice?
- How do I set up a new practice?
- How can I find out what running my own practice will be like before I actually own a practice?
- What about finding employees?
- How do I promote my new practice?

Why do you want to own a practice?

There are a number of perceived benefits to owning your own practice. The move from associate (which is akin to someone who rents their flat or house) to practice owner (someone who now owns the property) means more responsibility. Becoming a business owner will take over your life.

Hold this thought: practice ownership is a major, possibly lifetime, commitment.

Some dentists see buying a practice as an investment opportunity, something they can sell and make a profit on, or as an investment for their old age. For most people owning a practice is simply a way of earning (more) money.

Here are some of the benefits of practice ownership, mixed with a few words of caution.

- You might have more control over what you do and how you do it, but this is not always the case. If you work under the NHS you might not have any more control than you currently have in your present situation.
- There is a greater sense of self-determination: you hope you are going to be able to take the practice in the direction you want.
- You feel more independent and relatively free from the authority of others. There might not be a principal watching over you, but there will be others, the NHS, Care Quality Commission (CQC), private capitation scheme companies, a bank manager, for example.
- Your energies are channelled into working for your own interests and not those of others. This is true, but how much energy will be needed?

However, as with everything else in life, there are always drawbacks. Here are some of the reasons why owning a practice might not be such a good idea:

- you will certainly be taking financial risks with your money and with other people's (the bank's). If the finances don't turn out to be quite as rosy as you first predicted, you may be putting your family's future at risk
- you have the prospect of having to work (very) long hours, not only in the surgery to generate money, but also in the office managing the business
- sole responsibility for success or failure is yours; you hope your new practice is going to succeed, but how would you cope if it doesn't?
- even if you employ others to carry out these tasks, you will still have ultimate responsibility for finance, marketing and personnel. The buck stops with you!
- you probably won't enjoy the financial security that working in a larger and perhaps more well established practice offers, at least not in the early days.

My dentist (a practice owner) told me that these days most associates aren't interested in owning a practice, one reason being they are too expensive to buy. They prefer to acquire extra clinical skills and then work as a peripatetic associate, selling their skills to practices, presumably to the highest bidder. This gives the associate the freedom to move around, with no responsibility for staff, facilities management or any of the other things that go with practice ownership.

I have a dentist friend who used to be a practice owner, but they sold up, enhanced their clinical skills, and now work in several practices as an associate. They have said they are happy doing dentistry this way in preference to running a practice.

Who should *not* own a practice

If you have decided that owning and running a practice is what you want to do, even before you look for a practice to buy, or for premises to buy or lease in which you could set up a new practice, you need to assess your ability to cope with the inevitable pressures of running a business, and to answer several questions about yourself.

Are you self-disciplined? This is about being able to motivate yourself, stay on track and do what you have to do. Self-disciplined means being able to control your feelings and overcome your weaknesses. Are you level-headed or do you lose your head when things aren't going right? Do you know what your weaknesses are? You must ask yourself some tough questions.

- What are your personal strengths? Are you someone who likes to be in charge and gets thing done? Are you a team player?
- What are your personal weaknesses? Are you a poor listener? Are you arrogant and never listen to advice?

In the wider context, you should start to think about two other major questions:

- can you identify any opportunities that might give you an edge over the competition? Do you have additional clinical skills over and above those of other dentists?
- are there any (serious) threats that could (seriously) jeopardise your hopes and aspirations?

Don't do this on your own. Talk to friends and family, even work colleagues (without telling them the purpose of your questions), and build up a picture of how others see you. Try to eliminate any weaknesses, or at least work on minimising them.

Are you a doer or do you tend to let things drift? Some dentists simply aren't cut out to be practice owners. Your practice will never succeed unless you are in total control of everything that happens in it. You can employ a manager, a marketing manager, someone to do your PR etc. etc., but at the end of the day it is all about you being in control.

Do you have the unconditional, ongoing support of your family? Don't underestimate the importance of this. Relationships become very strained when things aren't going well. Selling the idea of practice ownership to your family might not be too difficult, but retaining their ongoing support and understanding through the difficult times is also going to be vitally important.

> The job you have, the mental toll it takes, and the personality you develop while in the job, all have an effect on your relationship with those around you. Changing your job from dentist to dentist *and* practice owner changes your relationships. Paradoxically, it also reveals the commitment of others to their relationship with you. Marriages can often fail because businesses fail.

How do you cope under pressure? At the moment you may be an associate, working hard and taking home more or less the same amount of money every month, more than enough to pay your mortgage, household bills, loans or leasing etc. You have no responsibilities for hiring or firing, for marketing or for anything to do with the management of the practice. Is your current situation stressful? If it is, it's going to get a lot worse as a practice owner. If it's not, how do you know if you'll be able to cope with the pressures of running your own show?

Would you be prepared to work 7 days a week if necessary? Long hours, not only in the surgery, but also seeing to everything else to do with managing a business. Hard work is going to be the name of the game.

Are you a leader or a follower? Being a practice owner means being a leader and, if you want to make a success of things, being an inspirational leader.

Can you make quick decisions when needed? Not only quick decisions, but the right decisions. You may well be able to make quick *clinical* decisions, but will you have the ability to make quick *management* decisions?

Are you a sticker or a quitter? Ownership can be a lonely place; when things get tough will you be prepared to see it through? Owning a practice is going to be a bumpy ride. Will you be all for handing the keys back the first time something goes wrong?

Can you learn from mistakes and take advice? This is fundamental to whether or not the practice is going to succeed or fail. If you don't or won't learn from your mistakes, you will continue making the same ones time after time, and that is not good.

Are you in good health? This is such an obvious factor, but one that perhaps is often overlooked. Skeletal problems or bouts of depression, no matter how mild, do not bode well.

If the answers to any of these questions are less than 100% positive, think twice about taking the plunge into ownership.

Hold this thought: practice ownership is not for the faint-hearted.

When is the best time for you to buy a practice?

There might never be a perfect time to buy a practice, but there might be a time when you should *not* buy a practice.

Consider your answer under three headings.

1. Personal.
2. Professional.
3. Financial (personal finance *and* the general economy).

Common sense should tell you that if your personal life is in turmoil, now is not the best time to start thinking about buying a practice. You wouldn't think of setting sail in a storm, would you?

Professionally you need to have sufficient clinical experience under your belt, so practice ownership is probably not something you should do until you've got the hang of successfully treating patients in a practice setting.

You will never know for certain if the time is right financially, you simply have to make a decision based on the current situation. One thing is worth pointing out, though, and that is that if your personal finances are not in good order it is going to be harder (if not impossible) for you to secure borrowing.

You are the only one who will know when the time is right. I would not even think about owning a practice unless all three of the above-mentioned factors are favourable.

Where's the best place to look for a practice?

Practices are most commonly advertised for sale in the dental press, on the Internet and on dental sales agent websites. However, there are other perhaps less obvious places where you can find out about practices that may not have yet come on to the open market.

- Your accountant is likely to know which of their practice-owner clients is contemplating retirement in the near future.
- Independent financial advisers will be talking to practice owners and so will know if any of them is thinking of selling or retiring.
- Dental company representatives hear all sorts of 'whispers' and might be able to put you on to practices that are coming up for sale.
- You can always talk to colleagues in other practices.

But in trying to find out what other people are up to, be careful that you aren't broadcasting your intentions.

Replying to an advert in one of the journals puts you in direct contact with the seller. However, there are some things you need to be aware of:

- confidentiality is very important for *both* parties
- the seller may have come up with the sale price him- or herself, so you need to find out whether or not it is a fair valuation and on what information the seller has based their asking price.

In much the same way as when you are looking to move house, you can get yourself on to practice agents' mailing lists, but you should be quite specific about the type of practice you are interested in otherwise you could end up being inundated with the particulars of every practice on their books.

What sort of practice do you want to buy?

NHS, private (fee-per-item or capitation), mixed, general or specialist? Remember that every type of practice carries its own opportunities and its own threats.

An NHS practice might have a certain amount of financial security and a semi-fixed income, but could potentially be difficult to expand.

Private practices are more prestigious, but will be at a premium in terms of purchase price. Capitation-based incomes could be more financially secure than a fee-per-item practice.

If you are not a specialist, you aren't going to look at buying a specialist practice.

Make sure you are aware of the threats to each type of practice.

What are your own personal pros and cons of owning each type of practice?

> The size of the property also matters. A colleague who owned a very successful specialist practice in the West End told me that when he was looking for somewhere in which to set up his new practice (initially one-surgery) he wanted a place that allowed for expansion. He was determined his practice would be successful, which it was.
>
> I found my practice by asking around. A friend of a friend eventually put me on to the one I bought. I'd asked reps (the ones I knew I could trust) if they knew of anywhere, and of course I'd scoured the ads in all of the dental press. It was a part-time practice when I bought it, but from day one I turned it into full time by simply being open 5 days a week. It also had an unused room which within a few months was converted into a hygienist surgery.

There are three options open to you with regards practice ownership, and three different scenarios.

- Buy an existing practice.
- Buy (into) the practice in which you currently work.
- Set up a new practice from scratch.

Each scenario will be explored later in more detail.

You should have thought about where in the country you want to work: what type of area you want your patient base to come from, city centre, suburban or rural? The location is important: where you are located influences your patient demographics. What type of patients do you want to treat?

Do you want to acquire a leasehold or freehold property? Leasehold means you will never own the building, but then again you don't have to finance the purchase of a building that you might not want. With freehold comes the full responsibility and cost of maintenance.

What determines the price of a practice?

Traditionally the selling (asking) price of a practice is based on what is known as the goodwill value, which is usually calculated as a percentage of the practice's gross fee income. Over the years goodwill values have fluctuated, but two phenomena have come into play, and hence the asking price for practices has increased.

- Large corporates entering the dental market. They were keen to build up a critical mass of practices and reap the economies of scale. They are usually better funded than individual dentists and are therefore likely to bid for and purchase practices for high prices.
- The 2006 dental contract, which brought more perceived stability to NHS practice gross incomes.

> During my time in practice, goodwill values were one day high and the next day low. At the time of writing I am hearing that goodwill is not worth anything. This situation can and probably will change.

There is a case for practice values being based not on turnover, but on a multiple of profit, as happens in other, non-dental businesses (the real world?). Practice owners with an above average profitable practice who are aware of this might therefore ask for more than its value based on goodwill. Owners of low profit practices are likely to stick to the old formula based on goodwill.

As well as buying the goodwill, you will be expected to buy fixtures and fittings, and the practice premises if they are freehold.

How do you know whether you are paying a fair price? You will need the services of a practice sales agent to give you a valuation. Don't rely on the vendor's valuation. (A specialist dental accountant will also tell you whether the business is viable.) Practice sales agents are specialised estate agents. Hopefully their knowledge of the dental market is going to mean that the seller receives a fair price and that you, as the buyer, pay a fair price. Going through a sales agent rather than buying via an advert may also smooth out the sale and purchase process. What does the final purchase price include? Don't assume it includes 'everything'.

As I've said, don't rely on the vendor's valuation. Remember that the asking price for dental practices obeys the law of supply and demand just like any other commodity. When supply exceeds demand, prices tend to be deflated; when demand exceeds supply, prices tend to be inflated.

Where and how do you find the finance?

Every purchase begins with the question of money, so very early on it is a good idea to talk to your bank manager about your future plans, even if at present they are no more than 'Well sometime, maybe in the next two to three years, I might be looking for a practice to buy.' At this stage you probably won't get any absolute guarantees or assurances from them about whether or not they will be prepared to lend you money at some time in the future. However, even at this very early stage you should be able to:

- give them an idea of the current asking price of a practice, and therefore how much you are likely to want to borrow
- demonstrate that you are aware how much any borrowings are likely to cost in terms of monthly repayments, not just at today's rates, but also if rates rise (as a rough guide, every thousand pounds you borrow at 5% over 25 years will cost you £6, or £4 per month interest only)
- outline your overall career plan, which includes buying a practice.

You need to develop a good relationship (if you haven't already got one) with your bank manager. If you put a great deal of the work into this now, when you eventually start seriously looking for a practice, hopefully obtaining the finance you require is not going to be too difficult. You must bear in mind that some banks and financial institutions are likely to want to see your business plan *before* they will even consider lending you any money. A well-researched and well-written business plan is going to be an important part of your future business, but even before then, it is likely to be an essential element in helping to secure finance for your enterprise. Before a bank asks to see your business plan, you need to know how to put one together.

Nowadays some businesses start up using non-bank-provided finance. Dentistry is on the whole a fairly traditional professional business, and while these sources of finance could be available, the majority of practice finance probably still comes from traditional sources, i.e. banks. However, wherever you look for finance, the same rigorous lending criteria used by banks should still be applied by the lender. This is as much for your benefit as for theirs.

Writing your (first) business plan

Buying or setting up your first practice means that you have decided to be a businessman or businesswoman, as well as a dentist. Dentists write treatment plans; people in business write business plans. The first step along the road to securing that all-important finance is to write your business plan.

A business plan essentially describes three elements of any business or practice.

- Operations: the premises in which the practice is located; equipment; employees; the services on offer.

- Finance: set-up costs; fixed and variable costs once the practice is up and running; minimal financial requirements.
- Marketing: how potential customers are going to be approached.

There are a number of sections to a business plan and they are all equally important. The following layout gives you an idea of what your business plan should eventually include.

1. Set the scene; attach a copy of your curriculum vitae (CV).
2. Set out your objectives, both personal and business.
3. Set out your analysis of the market.
4. Set out your approach to marketing your services.
5. Describe your future plans for researching and developing your services.
6. Set out your financial plan.
7. Give an accurate appraisal of the strength of the management of the practice.
8. Highlight any risks and problems that you have identified. Show that you have thought carefully about these and indicate how you propose to deal with them.
9. Finish your plan with your main conclusions, making sure that you leave the reader with a very positive impression.
10. Your plan should include an executive summary, which although mentioned last actually appears at the beginning. It is a complete, overall summary of every part of the plan.

The plan should be nicely bound and should have a front cover that shows:

- the title of the document, i.e. it is a business plan
- your name
- the name and location of the practice you are thinking of buying or setting up
- the date the business plan was written.

Set out below is an example of a business plan so that you can see the type of information it needs to contain, and to give you a better idea of the layout.

BUSINESS PLAN

Prepared by Dr A Tooth
For proposed practice purchase of *Super Dental Care, Anytown*
1 June 2015

EXECUTIVE SUMMARY

I have been an associate for 5 years and I am now ready to buy my first practice. I keep up to date with developments in clinical dentistry and have just embarked on a postgraduate training programme. Although I have no previous management experience I am taking steps to correct this.

The practice I want to buy is a busy National Health Service (NHS) practice in an excellent location with a great deal of passing trade. It currently turns over £X per annum. It is on the market for £X, which my advisers (*their names and who they work for*) think is a very reasonable asking price.

My objectives would be to increase patient numbers, to develop the services on offer, and to increase turnover and profitability.

This is a long-term investment and so gaining an excellent reputation in the area is going to be of paramount importance. Marketing will be backed up by excellent patient care.

BACKGROUND INFORMATION

I am a 28-year-old dentist. I qualified when I was 23 from London University; since then I have completed my foundation training and have worked full time as an associate in two very busy general NHS practices. I have attached my CV for additional information.

I started looking for a practice to buy over a year ago, but recently I have found one that interests me as a potential purchase. The current owner set up the practice from scratch in the early 1980s. It is a full-time, two-surgery NHS practice (only one of the surgeries is currently being used) in a converted 1970s three-bedroomed detached house, which is in the middle of a very large residential estate, with three more adjacent housing developments planned for the next couple of years. The practice is in a prominent position and is opposite a big parade of shops, two schools and a medical centre. There is a large (free) car park 2 minutes from the practice. The estate is 30 minutes' walk from the town centre. There is a good bus route between the estate and town (the nearest bus stop is 20 yards from the entrance to the practice). There are no other dental practices on the estate.

The practice has an NHS contract for £X. There is little or no private work carried out.

It is a retirement sale and the owner is asking £X for the goodwill, property, and the fixtures and fittings. My accountant thinks that the asking price is very reasonable. A local estate agent has indicated that the asking price for the property is average for a property of this type and condition.

I have had one viewing of the practice: the two surgeries need modernising; the reception area needs to be modernised; the outside of the building needs smartening up. The property needs to be surveyed and to have the electrics checked (it has not been rewired since it was built). The practice currently employs one full-time nurse and one full-time receptionist; both have been with the practice for around 4 years. The owner has said that both want to stay on after the practice has been sold.

I have walked past the practice on numerous occasions over the past 3 months, and at different times of day, and it is always busy. I would describe the practice as a 'family practice'.

MY OBJECTIVES

- To retain the existing NHS core of patients (currently 6000, but the current owner is not accepting new patients).
- To develop the range of clinical services.
- To attract new patients and therefore I will need to take on an associate (who can use the second surgery).

MY ANALYSIS OF THE MARKET

The town has a population of X, which is increasing because of new housing developments in the immediate area. The town has a thriving centre with many new businesses. There is low unemployment in the area. The town is a mixture of all social classes.

There are five dental practices, two of which are single-handed in the town. Two that are each worked by two dentists, and one that has four dentists (this one is on the High Street and is part of a national chain of practices). Three of the practices (both the two dentist ones and one of the single-handed ones) do not accept NHS patients. The nearest practice to *Super Dental Care* is 30 minutes on foot or 10 minutes by bus or car.

I have researched the demographics of the area.

HOW I INTEND TO MARKET MY SERVICES

All the other practices in the area advertise in Yellow Pages. I too will have an advert, stressing that I am accepting new NHS patients. I intend to also have a website.

I want my patients to be my main source of marketing, by providing them with a first class clinical service backed up by excellent customer care.

I have spoken to the local newspaper and they have said that they would be interested in me writing a short piece about my practice for them if and when I move in.

I intend to make myself known to local businesses, the schools and to the doctors in the medical centre.

FUTURE PLANS FOR DEVELOPING AND RESEARCHING MY SERVICES

I plan on providing quality NHS care, but will hope to increase the number of patients.

I will develop the range of services offered in line with up-to-date dental care and treatment protocols. I am a member of a study group and, together with my mandatory continuing professional development, keep up to date with developments in clinical dentistry. I have enrolled for a distance learning masters' degree in prosthetic dentistry; this will increase my clinical knowledge and give me a competitive edge over other practices in the area.

MY FINANCIAL PLANS

I have attached copies of financial projections (budget and cash flow) that my accountant has prepared. I have also included a copy of my personal income and expenditure, assets and liabilities (using the bank's pro forma).

I will need to borrow £X to purchase the property, goodwill and fixtures and fitting, plus an estimated £X for new equipment for one of the surgeries and reception, and general refurbishment (I will be able to provide more exact figures once the purchase has been finalised). I will also require £X as working capital. My accountant is confident that all borrowings and expenditure can be met from the projected practice income.

MANAGEMENT OF THE PRACTICE

I have no direct practice management experience. However, over the last year I have attended two practice management courses run by the British Dental Association; both courses were very informative.

I have been learning as much as I can about management from books and the Internet.

Initially I will manage the practice myself, but would hope in time to employ a professional practice manager to run the business.

My accountant and solicitor are both members of the National Association of Specialist Dental Accountants and Lawyers (NASDAL). They both fully understand the business of dentistry and are excellent advisers.

RISKS AND PROBLEMS

Central government funding of NHS practices is currently 'healthy'. This could change in the future.

There does not appear to be a great deal of direct competition from other practices in the area.

As with any NHS practice purchase, there could be problems having to undertake treatments that the current owner has failed to do but has been paid for. My solicitor will take every step to ensure that this is covered in the final sale contract.

I will do everything I can to increase and improve my managerial (people and financial) expertise.

CONCLUSIONS

Super Dental Care is currently a thriving NHS practice; it is in an excellent location with lots of passing potential patients; there is no competition in the area.

The asking price is both reasonable and affordable.

There is the potential to increase patient numbers and to expand into a two-surgery practice. Budget and cash-flow projections are positive. There is the potential to realise above average profit.

By putting together a business plan, even at this early stage, you will start to think like a businessman or a businesswoman, and a practice owner.

I spent almost half of my dental career working as an expert witness, and so I was used to writing reports for the legal profession. The book I wrote about the role of the expert includes a big chunk about how to write and set out a report, and why it is important that it ends up looking professional. Your business plan deserves the same respect.

Hold this thought: approach business ownership with the same professionalism as you give to your dentistry.

Common problems with business plans

A business plan is not like a treatment plan in that it does not describe what is to be done and when; it simply describes the business's goals. Your business plan should contain all of the elements that go to make up what you hope to achieve by being in business.

There are several common mistakes that people make when writing their business plan. The first mistake is that the financial information is often inadequate; this is probably the most important section of any business plan because any lender will want to know:

- when their money is going to be repaid
- the risk they are taking in lending the money.

All financial statements need to be able to stand up to rigorous scrutiny by an accountant. Don't think you can fudge the figures and then bluff your way past the accountant *and* the bank manager, and get away with it. You can't. Besides which, you're only fooling yourself if your figures are no more than wishful thinking.

Then, projections of business growth are often wildly over-optimistic and unrealistic. Again, we are back in the land of wishful thinking.

Hold this thought: it is better to exceed modest projections than fail to meet wildly optimistic ones.

Information is often left out because you have failed to read the question and have not done as the business plan format demands.

There is often a (very) poor understanding of marketing. The academic definition of marketing, according to the Chartered Institute of Marketing, is *The management process responsible for identifying, anticipating and satisfying customer requirements profitably.* Do you know how to market, or do your think it is just about selling?

Having put together a business plan, you fail to 'sell' it to, say, the bank. Although you might get someone else to help you write it, e.g. your accountant, you must be familiar with and understand everything it contains.

Optimism is often a major problem with business plans. Don't assume that the reader is going to be swept along by your enthusiasm; you will have to convince some cynics.

People fail to set their plan out logically and often the plan is not very well written. Simplify, but don't oversimplify; draft and redraft until it is right. You will have less difficulty convincing anyone of the viability of your proposal if you have taken the time and trouble to critically analyse every stage. Writing a good business plan takes time.

If writing a business plan seems a bit daunting, seek help from people with the relevant experience and knowledge and, most importantly, you should be prepared to listen to them. The major banks have business as well as personal customers, and part of the service they offer to businesses is help with drawing up a business plan. You should pick up copies of pro forma business plans from as many institutions as you can. They are all likely to be slightly different in one way or another, but when you have read them all you should be able to come up with your own template. Your business plan is personal to you.

Hold this thought: your business plan is important; it should also be personal.

3

The process of buying an existing practice

If nothing you've read so far has put you off becoming a practice owner, and you've decide that you want to buy an existing practice, and you think you've found the practice you want to buy, there are a number of questions you need to ask the vendor.

- Why are they selling? Perhaps an obvious question, but sometimes their reason(s) might not ring true.
- Has the practice made a consistent profit over a period of time, say the last 5 years? Where's the evidence?
- How many 'active' patients does the practice currently have? Where's the evidence?
- How many new patients does the practice attract per month? Where's the evidence?
- Are patient numbers growing, static or declining? Where's the evidence?
- Where is the nearest practice? Find this out for yourself.

> Holding on to the existing patients is a must for any new practice owner, so make sure that the current owner is not simply going to take the patients with them to some other nearby practice. I have come across this happening.

Question the current owner about their reasons for selling. Are they genuine? But there are also other things you will need to consider.

- If it is a retirement sale, think about how the patients will react to a younger, more up-to-date practitioner. Will they accept modern dentistry or will they leave to find someone else?
- How long has the current owner been there? If the current owner has only had the practice for a couple of years, and the turnover looks good and profitability looks promising, have they 'milked' the practice, leaving the next owner with no work?
- Where is the current owner going to work after they have sold up? Is there a risk of the patients following them?

You may think that you can buy a part-time practice and turn it into full time. Is this realistic? Has the current owner tried and failed?

> I know a dentist who bought a practice that had been 'milked' by the previous owners: high gross income, good profits, but not for the new dentist.
>
> A friend bought a single-handed, full-time practice. There wasn't enough work for him so he found another practice where he could work as an associate until his practice built up. His practice was then only open for 3 days a week. His practice contracted into a part-time practice and it didn't grow until he worked there 5 days a week. Your practice should be full time or no time.

When you eventually find the practice you want to buy, don't fall into the Pygmalion trap by falling in love with it at first sight, believing that you (and only you) can transform this little run-down, part-time, unloved, neglected practice (hence its very cheap purchase price) into the beautiful, state-of-the-art, full-time, everyone's favourite practice that you know lingers somewhere just beneath the surface.

Hold this thought: don't let your heart rule your head.

The recent profit and loss accounts may show a less than average profit, but the owner tells you that their accountant likes to reduce the profits to reduce their tax bill. This is fair enough, but is it true? Profit is linked to turnover and to costs; I would always pay closer attention to turnover because this is likely to be a more realistic reflection of a practice's earning potential. To some extent you can control your costs, but trying to build up a turnover could take years. You should always ask to see at least the last 5 years' profit and loss accounts. Always have your accountant look at them; don't pretend that you understand profit and loss accounts enough to know exactly what they might be telling you about the business.

> I spent a long time in dentistry and saw or heard various things that practice owners get up to when they were selling their practice. Trust between colleagues is all well and good, but when it comes to parting with your money, and probably lots of it, when you buy a practice, get everything tied down, wrapped up and bolted to the floor contractually.

Taking over existing staff can be fraught with difficulties. I recently heard of a dentist who bought a practice and was then saddled with a practice manager who was not supportive. The manager was eventually dismissed. To keep or not to keep existing staff is a tricky decision. If you are going to keep them, it is best to set your stall out right at the start so they are in no doubt about your vision for the practice.

Hold this thought: if you don't have a vision you risk the staff dictating how the practice develops, or not, as the case may be.

Hopefully the previous owner's patients will stay with you; you find there is thankfully a great deal of work to do; they are happy for you to go ahead with doing it. It can take some time to bring a cohort of patients' dental health up to your standard. This is all well and good, but when you've done all the work on these patients, are there others there for you to treat and from whom you can continue to earn your fees?

> After taking over my practice, it took me 2–3 years to sort the patients out (dentally), but then I found I'd run out of work, at least the bigger restoration jobs. Colleagues who have also bought practices have told me the same thing. So while you're treating all of these patients in your new practice, you should be thinking about how you are going to attract new ones. Marketing is an ongoing activity.

When you think about the practice you are eventually going to own, draw up a list of the 'must-haves' and 'nice-to-haves' for your practice. Must-haves include such obvious items as a dental chair and light, hand instruments, a steriliser, intra-oral X-ray equipment etc. Nice-to-haves are laser equipment, an OPT machine, opulent leather seating in the patients' waiting area! Set a realistic budget and stick to it.

> I didn't have a budget when I bought my practice. I got carried away buying equipment and setting up a second surgery, until I ended up borrowing more than I should have, and certainly more than I could comfortably pay back! Equipment salespeople are only there to sell you equipment. They aren't interested in how you are going to later pay for it. They will tell you that you will get 40% tax relief on any payments, which is true, but only if you make a profit!
> It took me 3 years of very hard work and countless sleepless nights to put things right.

No two practice purchases are the same; however, this section attempts to bring some clarity to what at times can be very complex and daunting processes. It also tries to highlight where and how the process can sometimes go (horribly) wrong.

There are some general comments to make (again) about buying or setting up a practice before the actual process begins. First, it is a major financial commitment: do not attempt to 'go it alone' by excluding your professional advisers from the process. Second, it is a life-changing event: make sure that you fully understand the risks you are taking and the commitment you are making. Before you buy any practice, get your own valuation.

These are the stages you will (should) go through when buying any practice.

- Contact the sales agent or vendor.
- Ask for a set of the profit and loss accounts going back several years, and anything else that could be relevant to the purchase and change of ownership.
- Speak to your accountant; tell them what you are planning to do.
- The accountant should then prepare financial forecasts for you based on information provided by the vendor.
- Meet with the bank manager and discuss the purchase. Hopefully they are going to approve the finance you need.
- Speak to your solicitor.
- Negotiate and make an offer to purchase.
- The accountant and solicitor should carry out due diligence on the business you are buying.
- Once the purchase has been agreed, discuss timings for the transfer with everyone concerned.
- Speak to the NHS and/or the capitation scheme provider if this is relevant.
- Meet the employees of your new practice.
- Plan refurbishment/re-equip/new employees etc.
- Finally, take over.

So, besides your 'team' (accountant, solicitor, practice sales agent), you are probably also going to have to talk to landlords, the NHS (in whatever shape or form), capitation plan providers, and perhaps government agencies, i.e. CQC. If you are buying the practice property you may have to engage a surveyor or even a structural engineer to establish whether the building is sound. You may want to radically improve or update the dental equipment and the building inside and out, in which case you are going to need dental equipment engineers, IT specialists, and a team of tradespeople, and probably an architect. You can see how buying a practice involves a great many people, but unless you get the right people working with you and for you, the whole experience can quickly turn into a nightmare.

You might have started to think about how long the whole purchase-and-moving-in-and-getting-the-practice-up-and-running process is going to take to complete. How long depends on a multitude of factors. Having worked out roughly how long it is likely to take, map out a timetable and try to stick to it. You must at least have some end-date in mind. Try to remain in control.

Hold this thought: don't try to short circuit the process when buying a practice.

What can go wrong during practice purchase?

Things can go wrong at any stage of the buying (or setting up) process, no matter what type of practice is involved.

There are, however, two factors that are common to all problems associated with practice acquisition: people and pounds.

- The vendor, their accountant and/or solicitor, or the sales agent, might be difficult and/or uncooperative (although why they might be is a mystery).
- Your accountant and/or solicitor might not have sufficient experience or expertise to handle the purchase. Consequently you pay over the odds for the practice and things end up taking longer than they should.
- The forecast figures don't add up or, worse, you and/or your accountant think you don't need them. The purchase goes ahead and you end up buying a non-viable practice.
- The NHS does not allow the vendor's NHS contract to be transferred to you.

- There are problems with employees, either retaining the ones you've inherited or finding suitable ones for a new practice.
- Refurbishment is not well managed; it runs over time and over budget.
- Patients are less likely to leave an NHS practice, but if you have bought a private practice, you find a significant number of patients aren't returning to see you.
- The vendor has not been treating their NHS and/or capitation scheme patients (supervised neglect). You are faced with having to do a great deal of work, possibly for nothing.

Who else will you have to involve?

You've found a suitable practice to buy; you've talked it over with your accountant, who is happy that the figures all add up; you've talked it over with your solicitor; the next thing to do is to ask the bank for the money. Most people have to borrow money to buy a practice; most people borrow from a bank. Don't believe that any bank is automatically going to lend to you.

Every bank has its own policy when it comes to lending money to dentists for practice purchase, but it is fair to say that there are certain baseline criteria and conditions that any bank manager will be looking to satisfy before agreeing to lend. Knowing what these criteria and conditions are beforehand is going to reduce the chance of your application being rejected. Make enquiries at your bank and try to uncover as much information as you can.

Before you approach your (or 'a' if you are not using your own bank) bank manager it is important that you talk the proposed deal through with your accountant, and with your solicitor if necessary. Your accountant is going to help you filter out the bad or risky purchases, and he or she will usually be able to put you in touch with the right bank, that is, one that understands the business of dentistry, and one that he or she knows looks upon dentists favourably. It is important that by the time you meet the bank manager you already have a good idea about how much you want (need) to borrow, how much the monthly repayments are going to be, and how much working capital you are going to require. Don't waste the bank manager's time by approaching them *before* you've thoroughly explored the proposition with your accountant.

Let's assume that you have never met this particular bank manager before (even if you are using your own bank, you might be meeting a new manager). What things are they going to be looking for or at? The first thing they are going to do, and this is human nature, is to assess you as a person. Do you look the part? Do you come across as knowing what you are talking about? Presenting yourself dressed in torn jeans (even if they are designer!) tee shirt and trainers does not send the right message.

The bank manager will also want to know:

- whether you know what you are getting into
- whether you can run a practice. This might be extremely difficult to ascertain because the majority of associates have had no experience of practice management. By the time they become practice owners it is too late to discover that they really aren't good at business.
- if you are any good at people management. You are not going to be able to run the practice without the help of others. If you are no good at managing people, it does not matter how good you are as a dentist or how swish your practice looks, you will probably not have the support workers to enable you to treat your patients
- the state of your personal finances. The bank manager will want to see *all* your personal financial commitments, personal bank statements, credit card statements etc. If they see, or even suspect, that you are not capable of managing your personal finances, they are unlikely to let you loose with any more money. You will usually be expected to fill in an Asset and Liability/Income and Expenditure form (*see* Figure 3.1). Hopefully the left-hand side will be more than the right-hand side
- whether after having paid out everything for the business, together with what it takes to support your lifestyle, there is a comfortable margin. The bigger the margin, the better
- what you are bringing to the practice by way of specialist skills and expertise

INCOME AND ASSETS	EXPENDITURE AND LIABILITIES
Your monthly income/drawings from practice. Your spouse's/partner's income. Any other income	*All* household and personal expenditure
Value of your property(ies)	Outstanding mortgage and/or loans secured against property(ies)
Other assets, e.g. savings, shares, life policies (surrender value)	Outstanding debts

Figure 3.1 Asset and Liability/Income and Expenditure form

- what the practice will be losing. If the current owner leaves will most of the value of the practice be walking out of the door with them?
- whether or not you are a bona fide dentist and are on the Dental Register.

The above can be summarised in the acronym CAMPARI, which stands for:

- Character; yours and everything about you.
- Ability; what do you know about running a business?
- Margin; how much is the bank going to make?
- Purpose; can you prove your reason to the bank?
- Amount; can you justify the amount you are asking for?
- Repayment; will you be able to meet the repayments?
- Insurance; what security are you able to offer?

Having successfully negotiated this first hurdle, the bank manager is next going to look at the particulars of your case and make an assessment of the risks (from the bank's point of view, but ultimately from yours as well) and whether or not you have fully considered them. They will want to know:

- after financing of the purchase, how much needs to be spent on updating equipment, renovating the property etc.
- in the case of an NHS practice, whether there are going to be any claw-backs
- what is happening to the vendor. Where are they going to be working? Is there the possibility that they could set up nearby?
- your employees are a vital element of the practice. Are any of the current employees staying on and are any of them key to your future plan? The current owner might have a team that has been together for several years, but if there are doubts about whether one or more of them will be staying, this could prove to be a risk
- if the projected income is sustainable. You should be slightly pessimistic about any financial projections and not get carried away with the belief that your income is only going to go one way, and that is up
- the EBITDA, that is earnings before interest, tax, depreciation and amortisation. (Amortisation means gradually paying off a debt.) EBITDA is basically the profit of the business *after* drawings but *before* borrowing costs, taxes and 'non-cash' items such as depreciation of equipment and amortisation of goodwill have been taken into account. Your accountant should help you work this out
- whether the practice is worth what you are paying for it. Is the value of the goodwill accurate? Is the practice in a good location? How many potential patients pass its door each day (footfall)? Your accountant should have helped you establish that you are not paying over the odds. The bank manager is more likely to give credence to a valuation from an accredited and recognised practice sales agent as opposed to a valuation that has been dreamt up by the vendor who just wants to see how much he or she can get
- what you know about the area you are buying into. Have you done your homework? Have you drawn up a business plan and a marketing plan that seriously analyse the competition,

demographics (this information is easy to find on the Internet), the wider picture of central government and their future plans for dental healthcare and services etc.

- the structure and terms of the proposed borrowing
- whether you have got the right advisers behind you.

The above can be summarised using the acronym PARTS, that is purpose, amount, repayment, terms and security, which will all have to be right for the person (you) *and* for the bank. You will notice that all of these questions are the ones I highlighted earlier.

Knowing how banks operate when they are assessing a borrowing proposal is useful inside information. You should have done your homework and have the answers to any question the bank manager might throw at you.

Hold this thought: like all successful generals, you need advance information about the terrain on which you're likely to be fighting.

The bank manager will see their role in the practice purchase process (and beyond) as being one where they:

- ask the right questions
- give practical advice
- make sure that the proposed purchase has been well thought through
- see that all the risks have been identified and steps taken to minimise their impact.

They should in turn only be lending (responsibly) to:

- creditworthy people
- those who have a track record of sound personal financial management
- people whose future income is sustainable.

As long as you can satisfy all of the above criteria you are unlikely to encounter any problems raising finance. You should, however, be aware that banks will only lend to dentists who have done their homework and whose financial projections stack up. The days when a dentist could simply present themselves at the bank manager's door and be guaranteed a loan to buy a practice are long gone.

If the bank won't lend you as much as you were hoping for, they will usually have a very good reason for not letting you have more. Don't then go looking elsewhere for this extra money; you risk putting yourself under unnecessary financial pressure.

> Over the course of my dental career I had a number of bank managers: some were good; some were bad; some were indifferent. What makes a good bank manager? It is not the one who hands out loads of money; it is the one who understands your business and provides constructive help and support when you need it.

The role of your accountant

You probably already have an accountant, but if you are currently working as an associate, it is unlikely that they have so far given you any significant business advice. They may not actually know a great deal about the business of dentistry. Now is when you discover their limitations. However, using a specialist dental accountant should help you maximise the income and profitability of your practice by:

- comparing your financial results with local and national averages to identify areas in which you could improve
- improving its profitability by reviewing fee rates, the organisational structure of the practice, its management, and by looking at cost-effective practice finance packages
- minimising your tax liability by ensuring all expenses are claimed and by reviewing the timing of the year-end. This might be basic but they are very necessary accountancy services
- assisting with your record keeping and payroll and providing advice on efficient and cost-effective bookkeeping systems

- ensuring all tax return information is correctly completed and filed
- checking superannuation contributions and advising on alternative pension options to maximise retirement income.

A specialist dental accountant should give you better advice and support than an accountant who only has one dental client, i.e. you!

Returning to practice purchase, the accountant's role is to:

- interpret, analyse and evaluate the practice accounts, which at this stage will tell you two things:
  - the level of turnover and profit
  - whether the asking price is fair. (Don't think that you are qualified to work this out for yourself.)
- prepare financial forecasts, which will determine whether or not the potential purchase, at the price the vendor is asking, is going to be financially viable for you. It is important that you find this out now, not after you have signed the contract! Financial forecasting will help you
- put you in contact with banks who are likely to fund the purchase on favourable terms
- perform a due diligence examination of the practice. It is critical that you know that what you are thinking of buying is what it claims to be. If it is not, you can go back to the vendor with a revised offer. Your solicitor is also likely to be involved with performing due diligence. If you haven't got a solicitor, your accountant should be able to introduce you to a specialist dental solicitor
- at a later date, and if relevant, help you with your bid for an NHS contract.

Once you have decided to buy a practice it is important that you keep in touch with your accountant because they provide much needed advice and support, as well as introducing you to the right people.

Due diligence is about looking closely at the business's records: financial statements; contracts with employees, suppliers, customers; insurances etc. For a buyer it is about asking the right questions and then looking in the right places for the answers.

Hold this thought: accountancy largely deals with things that have already happened, but a good accountant should be helping you look to the future.

The role of your solicitor

A specialist dental accountant is an essential member of your business team, as is a specialist dental solicitor. A specialist solicitor can give you advice in a number of important areas.

- Business purchases and sales.
- Practice arrangements.
- Expense sharing agreements.
- Property ownership.
- Employment law issues.

With specific reference to practice purchase, a solicitor will:

- assist with and draw up the terms of the deal, for example:
  - confidentiality
  - exclusivity
  - restrictive covenants
- perform due diligence. Any major issues need to be identified early on so that any indemnities, warranty protection or retention of part of the purchase price can be inserted into the agreement

- advise on and draw up the sale agreement. The vendor will want an agreement that minimises their post-sale obligations and liabilities, while you will want to ensure that you are covered for anything that might go wrong with the practice post purchase, such as:
  - claw-back by the NHS
  - patient charges
  - indemnities for contractual obligations
  - transfer of the property
- liaise with your bank, to ensure that:
  - the bank's requirements are met throughout the purchase
  - funds are released as soon as they are needed at completion
- liaise with your accountant to ensure that the transaction works from a tax planning point of view
- employment, so that the transfer of any employee contracts is properly carried out
- work with the NHS to ensure that the contract (the patients) are transferred to you
- post purchase, a solicitor will:
  - register the transfer of the title with the Land Registry if it's a freehold property you've bought
  - make sure that the necessary stamp duty is paid
  - confirm with the bank that all of their requirements have been met
  - advise if any disputes arise.

Once you have taken ownership of your practice, you must have a solicitor to advice you on all legal matters to do with your business. You may also want to use the services of other dental organisations for your day-to-day legal advice, but having a knowledgeable solicitor on hand as a back-up is never a bad thing.

> I had a brilliant solicitor for all of the time I was a practice owner. He had a very sharp mind, was quick to see the problem, and know how to solve it in one hit. Don't end up with someone who is simply lining their own pockets.

The role of other professionals

There are other professionals who you may have to involve when you are buying a practice, mainly to do with the property, for example:

- if you are buying a freehold property:
  - a surveyor, to tell you whether the asking price is a true reflection of its value, and to uncover any faults (major or minor) with the fabric of the property
  - a structural engineer if there are any concerns about the foundations
  - an architect, if you are contemplating any structural alterations
  - a building contractor to cost out repairs or any planned alterations
- if you will be leasing the property:
  - a surveyor to tell you whether the rent you are being asked to pay is fair.

> When I bought my practice the bank insisted that their surveyor had a look at the property I was buying; this was to both value it and to help me cost out the refurbishment work I planned. Part of the building also showed signs of movement so I had to engage a structural engineer to look at this. Fortunately he deemed the building safe and unlikely to move in the future. (He was right.)

Post-purchase: working with building contractors

The vendor is not going to allow you to make any alterations or changes, no matter how small, to their practice before you have exchanged contracts and ownership has legally passed to you.

Whether you are simply intending to give your new practice a lick of paint or go for a full refurbishment, then as soon as ownership is yours, you must have everything and everyone ready for the off. Remember, any time lost between you taking over the practice and you starting work is costing you money. You are therefore going to need all your project management skills during this period.

You should find all of the builders, electricians, plumbers, heating engineers, painters and decorators etc. well in advance of when you want them to start work for you.

What is the best way of finding good, reliable tradespeople?

- Personal recommendation from someone whose opinion you trust is usually a good place to start.
- Use local people or firms.
- Only use people and firms that are members of the respective governing body, e.g.
  - electrical contractors – look for 'NICEIC' or 'ELECSA' registration
  - gas engineers – look for 'Gas Safety Trust' (formally CORGI) registration
  - builders – look for members of the Federation of Master Builders
  - window fitters – look for 'FENSA' registration.

You shouldn't think about using tradespeople who are not local because should there be a problem after the work has been completed you might have difficulty getting them to travel back to put it right. Having said that, the same can also happen if you use a local firm.

Building contractors often subcontract their work, which means that although you might meet and talk through the proposed work with the head person, the people who actually do the work might come from much further down the food chain.

> My wife and I had a new bathroom fitted a few years ago. We went to a national DIY and home improvements retailer thinking that they would do a good job. We later found out that this company subcontracts all of the bathroom work, and then discovered that the subcontractor also subcontracted the work. To cut a long story short, the bathroom we had fitted was not fit for purpose and it had to be redone. We successfully sued the national DIY company and got the bathroom we wanted. TV consumer programmes endlessly highlight the shortcomings of tradespeople. Just because these people are working in a dental practice does not mean they suddenly turn into angels.

It is always a good to know in advance how things should be done even if someone else will actually be doing the work for you. To help you here is the normal order of work in a property refurbishment.

- Carry out an inspection of the property with your builders etc. to determine what work is needed. Hopefully the vendor will allow you to do this before purchase is completed; if not, you will have to wait until after completion. It is at this stage that you must obtain quotations for all the necessary work. Some contractors may only be willing to give you an estimate; there is a difference between an estimate and a quotation:
  - an estimate is the likely price that will be charged for specified work
  - a quotation is a formal statement of the cost of a job.

On the surface there appears to be little difference between the two terms. Try to get an estimate of the maximum likely cost in the hope that it will end up being less, and then get it in writing. Never work to a verbal estimate. A written quotation is your safest option. In the same way as your patients have to trust you when you give them estimates, you will have to trust your contractors. But don't rely on one estimate, get at least three. And finally, when you've decided who to use, get everything set out in a watertight contract.

You might have to show the estimates to a lender.

- Rip out all the old fixtures and fitting, wiring, plumbing, walls, doors, flooring etc.
- Carry out all building work. This could include any external work, for example to the roof, or fitting new windows.

- Carry out the first fix of the electrics, plumbing etc. A first fix means running all cabling in and on walls, under floors, in the ceiling, and installing the back boxes for sockets and switches, as well as running all piping for the plumbing.
- Any plasterwork is then completed, which means walls are plaster boarded and skimmed. Door casings are fitted.
- Skirting boards and door architraves are then fitted.
- A first inspection can be carried out at this stage. The electrics, plumbing etc. should be tested.
- Doors fitted.
- Painting and decorating done.
- Second fix of electrics and plumbing, which means fitting sockets and switches, and radiators. Contractors must be very careful not to damage work already completed.
- Lay new flooring.
- Final inspection carried out.

Once you know the extent of the work needed, set it all out on your project management Gantt chart (*see* Figure 3.2 below). You might choose to project manage the work yourself, or you could leave it to the contractors to sort things out between themselves. This second option can be risky. You could do a little of both. Have the lead contractor draw up a Gantt chart, which you then discuss with them. Insist on periodic site meetings so you can check on progress and so that you can monitor the budget.

There has not been one house makeover programme on the television where the homeowners have not gone over time and over budget!

I wanted an extension added to my house. The great thing about being a dentist is that you come across so many different professions and tradespeople during the normal course of your work, and so I asked one of my patients who ran a building firm to give me a quote. I knew this chap, his wife, his son, and his business partner and his wife and kids. I knew I could trust them. Anyhow, I got a quote and the work was completed to a very high standard as per schedule. What I didn't know was that the two business partners were also architects who liked the hands-on side of property development. They project managed the whole thing themselves.

Hold this thought: having set your own timescales and budget, stick to them.

	Period 1	Period 2	Period 3	Period 4	Period 5	Period 6	Period 7	Period 8	End date
Task 1									
Task 2									
Task 3									
Task 4									
Task 5									
Task 6									
Task 7									
Task 8									
Task 9									

Figure 3.2 A basic Gantt chart

Project management

If the practice you are thinking of buying needs a great deal of refurbishment and/or building work, or if you are setting up a cold squat (i.e. a new practice), you are going to have to know how to manage the whole project. In essence, project management is about coordinating people, their activities, time and money: it is the process of planning, organising and managing resources to bring about the successful completion of a project's goals and objectives. The primary challenge of any project is meeting deadlines and constraints in terms of time and money.

Learning how to manage a project is going to prove an invaluable skill in the period before and after practice purchase.

A useful project management tool is the Gantt chart, which is basically a bar chart that allows the key stages of a project to be plotted against time. A Gantt chart enables you to visually coordinate and control everything that you and others must do as part of buying or setting up a practice.

To use this chart, define what each task is, how long it should take to complete, and plot each one against the horizontal timescale. Some tasks will probably overlap each other and some tasks will not be able to commence before others have been completed. Build in some leeway so that deadlines and the end date are not put under too much pressure. Things always take longer than you think, and not everyone will give your project the same importance and high priority as you have.

Hold this thought: don't underestimate the complexity of all of this – it represents a major challenge.

4

Incorporation

You might have already discussed incorporation with your accountant and solicitor, but if you haven't, the question of whether or not you incorporate your new practice, or even if you are thinking of incorporating a practice you've owned for a while, needs careful consideration.

The vast majority of dental care and treatment in the UK is carried out in dental practices, which come in all shapes and sizes. Practices are usually owned by a dentist or dentists and run as small businesses, either under the dentist's name or, if the practice has a business name, as 'Dr A trading as Nice Dental Care'. Prior to the Order to amend the Dentists Act 1984 there were 28 Dental Bodies Corporate (DBC), but in July 2005 this all changed and since then any corporate body can now carry on the business of dentistry provided they satisfy the requirements in relation to directors of bodies corporate as set out in Section 43 of the amended Dentists Act. The majority of directors of a DBC must be registered dentists or registered DCPs or a combination of dentists and DCPs.

The advantages and disadvantages of operating your practice as a sole trader or as a DBC lie outside the scope of this book; all I will say is that you must seek independent legal and professional advice before you proceed with any change to the legal status of a practice.

However, here are just a few of the things you should be aware of if and when you ever think about incorporation.

- The new company (Nice Dental Care Limited) is a separate legal entity, and is not simply Dr A with a tax-saving wrapper around them.
- When the move from personal to company takes place, assets and liabilities have to be legally transferred from one to the other. This becomes complicated where existing third party finance is concerned. Valuations, for example of goodwill, will have to be carried out.
- Primary care trusts will have to be involved if you have an NHS contract.
- Employee contracts, terms of employment etc. will have to be transferred to the new company.
- Your current CQC registration will have to stop and a new application for registration in the name of your new incorporated practice submitted.

Any registrations for any organisation will have to cease and new ones be taken out. Incorporation will take up a great deal of your time and/or the time of other people whom you are paying, so it will cost you money.

Someone I know had set up a limited company a number of years ago because at the time it was the most tax-efficient thing to do. When they retired they decided they no longer needed the company. They had to legally transfer the assets (property) of the company back to personal ownership. This was a fairly simple and straightforward process, but it nevertheless had to involve an accountant, a solicitor, and a fair amount of money.

Staying where you are: buying (into) the practice in which you currently work

On the face of it, this may seem like taking the line of least resistance, the easiest option of all – better the devil you know.

The practice principal might offer you a partnership or give you the opportunity to buy the practice outright.

What are the perceived advantages of becoming a partner?

- You stay where you are.
- You continue to treat the same patients.
- You more or less know what your income is going to be, but not necessarily the costs.
- You know the employees.
- You know the practice – warts and all.

However, before you jump at the chance to own your own practice, albeit perhaps only a share of one, ask the principal:

- What am I actually buying? Is it just the goodwill (or debt) or is it a share of the property (if it is freehold), fixtures and fittings etc?
- What are my rights regarding selling my share if I decide to leave?
- Who is responsible for funding the replacement of equipment etc?
- What arrangements will there be with regard to practice expenses?
- Will I have a say in recruitment, practice development, marketing, and management?

If you are offered a partnership you should always seek advice from your accountant and solicitor.

The owner of the first practice I worked in as an associate had three associates. It soon became apparent that the owner had financial problems (these things are difficult to keep quiet) and so offered us all partnerships. I showed the offer to my financial adviser who told me not to accept. The partnership offer was based on fanciful financial projections. The other two accepted; I declined and went in search of another associateship.

If the principal offers you the chance to buy the whole practice, approach this in the same way as if you know nothing at all about the practice. (*See* Chapter 2 *Do you really want to own a practice?* and Chapter 3 *The process of buying an existing practice.*)

Setting up from scratch

In the 1980s dental magazines were full of articles by dentists who had set up what is known as a 'cold squat', i.e. they set up a new practice from scratch. Often these articles gave the reader the impression that starting your own practice in this way was very easy and that no matter what you did it was always going to be a roaring success. No doubt some of them were successful, but would it be wise to try to do it today?

The advantages of setting up from scratch are:

- you probably have more freedom regarding the location
- you probably have more freedom when it comes to the layout
- you probably have more freedom to equip the practice the way you want
- you are not paying anyone for goodwill.

There are, however, a number of significant drawbacks, for example:

- you will have to invest a great deal of time, money and effort attracting patients
- your income will start at zero and might take months, even years, to reach your breakeven point, let alone return a healthy profit.

If you decide that you prefer to start from scratch rather than buying an existing practice, there are really only three things you need to seriously think about, which are location, location, location.

Hold this thought: set your practice up in the wrong area and you run the risk of it never reaching its full potential.

It might be very appealing, creating your own practice from nothing; moulding it, getting everything just as you want it. You are, however, going to need a great deal of drive, enthusiasm, perseverance, dedication, stamina, vision and money.

You will only be able to set up an NHS practice if there is a need for one in the area, and even then it is dependent on the favour of the local NHS managers. It is easier therefore to set up a private general practice from scratch.

If you decide to set up a private general practice from scratch, you will need to re-read Chapters 2 and 3, and the whole of Sections III, IV and V.

Setting up a specialist private practice

I have not included setting up an NHS practice here because at the time of writing I was not sure dentists did this any more.

Whether you plan to set up a private practice or a specialist private practice, the process is more or less the same.

However, setting up a specialist practice is not just about setting up a practice, it is also a long-term exercise in marketing, not only marketing your clinical expertise, but also yourself as someone in whom your colleagues are prepared to put their trust.

The majority of private specialist practices are operated by dentists who:

- possess a relevant postgraduate qualification in their chosen specialism
- have a proven track record of clinical expertise
- accept the majority of their patients by referral.

Setting up a specialist private practice, one that is going to be a long-term success, is going to be very difficult (if not impossible) unless you fall into the first two of these categories.

Provided you have the necessary qualifications and clinical expertise, how do you go about setting yourself up in specialist practice?

You could begin by renting a surgery in an already well-established specialist practice, or even in a general practice. There would be minimal set-up costs associated with this approach. If it doesn't work out, you probably wouldn't end up losing too much money; only your pride would suffer.

Whether you adopt this toe-in-the-water approach or go all out and set up a practice, you will need to build up your source of referrals from colleagues. You can do this by:

- writing to all the dentists in your area telling them:
  - who you are
  - where you will be working
  - what you are proposing to do, i.e. accept referrals
  - the type of treatment on offer
  - the terms under which their patients will be treated, i.e. privately
  - how they should refer patients to you
- hold an open day or evening when dentists you hope are going to refer patients to you can view your practice. Impress them with the quality of the facilities; let your employees talk to them so that the dentists see that the whole practice is a very well run and highly professional operation
- offer to talk at local dental meetings
- start a study group
- write articles in the dental press.

You are going to have to work hard on your marketing and on your customer care. Don't become so self-absorbed with your clinical skills that you forget that you are treating people, and forget that it is your customer care that really matters.

Some specialists work in a number of practices, perhaps because there isn't enough work in one area, or maybe that's how they prefer to work.

Making yourself well known in the dental world might not seem at first sight to be a way of attracting patients; however, it can be an effective strategy. I will explain.

Being on the speakers' circuit and/or writing articles etc. imparts a certain authority and status upon a person. That person then becomes someone with whom other dentists want to be associated, ideally by referring patients. The specialist can advertise what they've been getting up to outside of the practice in their promotional material within the practice, which is seen by patients, who in turn think it is nice to be treated by someone who must be very well respected within the profession. It is a circular and self-feeding process.

You should now re-read Chapters 2 and 3, and the whole of Sections III, IV and V.

New build

I imagine it is many a practice owner's dream and ambition to design, build and then work in what is truly their own practice: to not be confined by the constraints of previous designs and configurations; free to build a state-of-the-art facility.

Building your own practice literally from scratch really is a long-term plan and one that has a much longer lead-in time than any of the other options open to would-be practice owners. It will call on all of your managerial and project management skills.

The first thing to say is that it is probably not an option for an NHS practice, so a new build by default has to be a private practice, either general or specialist, or perhaps a mixture of both.

Is it something for one person to take on, or is it something that needs several dentists or DCPs to be involved in? Going it alone is one option, or you might put together a consortium of like-minded clinicians and/or investors. You will certainly need an accountant, a solicitor, a bank manager, an architect, and be able to work with planning departments, as well as other agencies.

I think it unnecessary to go through all possible scenarios; for now all you need to think about is the following.

As part of the planning stage (not the obtaining of planning permission) decide what it is you want to achieve. This is not simply 'a new practice': you must be very specific. Consider the location, size, number of surgeries, reception area(s), offices, demographics, finance, timescales etc. You might already have a practice, so what are you going to do with that?

Next, think about all of the resources you will have to gather together. At this early stage this largely means pounds and people (some of the people were mentioned earlier). Later on it will be builders and contractors.

Once you are ready to go ahead with building, you then will have to get these people to work together smoothly and to the best of their ability as part of a team to do the work.

Finally, you (and any business partners) must monitor, review or measure the progress of the build in relation to the plan, and take steps to correct things if they wander off course.

I have no personal experience of a dental new build, but I do have experience of a medical new build, well almost, as the plans were scrapped when things were well advanced through a lack of money. This was after the doctors had spent a great deal of time, energy and money. The plan was ambitious, but in the end the doctors had to settle for a major refurbishment of their existing premises.

For most dentists, moving into or taking over an existing building is usually the way of things, but a new build, given the right set of circumstances, could be a possibility.

7

How can I find out what being my own boss will be like?

Before you look for a practice, do as much research as you can and gain as much knowledge and background information about what running a business actually entails.

- Talk to practice owners, not only ones who appear successful, but also to ones who have perhaps made the odd mistake along the way. It is better to learn from other people's mistakes rather than make them yourself. People are often shy about revealing their mistakes, but some are willing to share them with others. People who say they have never made a mistake have probably never done anything!
- Find a mentor, a practice owner, to guide you.
- Talk to colleagues who are already practice owners. You should find out about the process of practice purchase (if they have bought recently), especially the pitfalls and problems. You also want to know something about how they manage their practice. Listen intently to what they say and form your own opinion as to whether they are doing it well, doing it badly, or not doing it at all.
- Speak with your accountant to get the inside track on the world of dental business.
- Speak with your solicitor to gain an insight of the legal minefield you'll have to navigate.
- Find out about business planning, have a go at writing a business plan for your imaginary practice.
- Consult your bank.
- Speak to local or regional business organisations and see what start-up help is available. The government might have agencies where you can obtain some free advice and support. Forget any ideas that the business of dentistry is unlike other businesses; all businesses are the same, so if there is advice out there, especially if it is free, use it.

Hold this thought: be prepared to not only listen to advice, but to also take it.

The greatest source of 'learning' is going to be the practice in which you are currently working. The practices that deliver the best patient care are the ones that are very well managed. Therefore, if you are fortunate enough to work in a very well managed practice, find out how they do it. If you are unlucky and you work in a very badly managed practice, work out why they are getting it wrong and what you would do differently to put things right. The majority of practices lie somewhere in the middle and so you will always be able to find examples of good and bad management in your current practice.

It is always easy to criticise what someone else does or how they do it; the key is to find out *why* they do it and in particular why they do it that particular way. So while you are observing the management of your current practice try to find out why things are done the way they are.

Having read books about management and dental practice management, you should now be in a position to not only judge the standard of what is being done, but also to recognise what is *not* being done. Again, find out why.

> It was not until years after when I was managing my own practice that I came to realise how badly managed were the practices I'd worked in previously. So-called practice managers who, when pressed, would not have any idea how to manage; no forward planning of any sort; no sense of anyone working as part of a team.

Initial thoughts about recruitment

It may be some time off, but you should give some thought to how you are going to recruit employees, how many you are going to need, and the personal qualities, qualifications and experience you will be looking for. As a rule of thumb:

- employ people with the best qualifications and the most experience you can find and can afford
- try to only employ those who are committed to providing excellent patient care and service. Patient care can, however, be taught; it is the employee's attitude and personality that is key
- don't 'over-employ', i.e. employ more people than you need in case someone might be off sick.

> I know a single-handed practitioner who employs a full-time nurse, a full-time receptionist, and a spare full-time nurse 'just in case'. His 'just in case' nurse provides cover if ever one of his other two staff is off work because of illness. I asked him, how often does this spare nurse have to cover for one of the others? About 5 or 6 days a year, was their reply. A quick calculation told me that he was paying around £3,000 per day for these 5 or 6 days of cover, and for his supposed peace of mind. I'd say he'd be better off using an agency nurse, or perhaps soldiering on each day with one staff. Surely he wasn't going to lose three thousand pounds in one day by just having one member of staff on hand. It might be hectic, but it is doable.

It is easier to take on who you want when setting up from scratch because you can choose your own employees. If you are buying an existing practice you might be asked or expected to take on the existing employees under the Transfer of Undertaking (Protection of Employment) Regulations (TUPE). You should ask the current owner to provide you with details of each individual's employment record, which you should examine closely for:

- sickness record (what level of sickness is acceptable?)
- disciplinary records (don't take on trouble)
- qualifications (signifies commitment)
- training (both previous and planned).

Don't saddle yourself with employees who are likely to be a problem. Seek legal advice if you are unhappy about taking anyone on. One of the major problems with inheriting someone else's employees is getting them to do things the way you want them done. You will need to talk to them, explaining that you are now in charge and that from now on things are going to be done differently. If any of them are unhappy with this, maybe now's the time for them to look for another job.

If you are the 'new boy' in your new practice and the other employees have been together for a while and formed their own friendship group, just be aware that this could lead to you feeling excluded.

> When I took over my practice I also took over the receptionist. She knew all of the patients, which I obviously didn't, so she'd chat away to them like she was at a coffee morning or something. I thankfully had taken my own nurse, a girl I'd worked with for two and a half years, so I didn't feel like the complete outsider.

Promoting yourself and the practice: the early days

Your marketing campaign should start as soon as you have ownership. (It could have started before that if you were 100% certain that the purchase would happen.) Ways of marketing your practice and of making people aware that something new and exciting is happening in their area include:

- recruiting employees from the local area – they can help you spread the word
- making yourself known to local businesses – visit them and leave your business card
- encourage your friends to talk about you and your practice on social networking sites

- create your own blog and talk about the trials and tribulations of owning a practice
- contact the local newspaper and get them to write a feature about you and the practice – free advertising.

Don't waste money on flyers or adverts in newspapers; takeaways and businesses desperate for customers do that, but not successful dental practices.

You basically want to create a 'buzz' in the local area, with everyone talking about and showing an interest in you and your practice (but only for the right reasons). Wouldn't it be good if within weeks of taking over you had more patients and work than you could handle? A nice problem to have.

The vendor is unlikely to have let you have access to individual patient records pre-purchase. Once the patients are yours you should go through the records building up a profile of the patients; where they are from; their gender; how old they are. Before you even put in an offer for the practice you should have carried out some form of demographic analysis of the area you are moving into to get at least a rough idea of the economics, characteristics, employment/unemployment level and potential for future growth.

Knowing where your patients are from and therefore how far they travel is important. If you have bought from a dentist who has practised there for a number of years, it is likely that some of the patients are second generation, that is, they have moved away from the family home (to work or to university) and might therefore be travelling a long way (back home) to see their dentist. Are they going to continue doing this? Do you want patients who travel a long way to see you, and who will probably expect, if not demand, single-visit treatment? It is flattering to have these travellers, but not always practical in terms of providing them with comprehensive dental care.

The age distribution of the patients is important. A practice with a predominately elderly patient base is not going to lend itself to cosmetic dentistry as easily as a younger patient base is likely to.

Once you have bought the practice you might want to change the patient demographics by focusing your marketing campaign on attracting specific groups of patients.

Summary

Buying your first practice is an enormous step that will inevitably bring about some massive changes in your life, not just professionally but personally. The commitment you have to make to ensure that your practice is a success should not be underestimated. It may seem that I have merely thrown lots of questions at you without providing many of the answers; unfortunately, that's how it is. You are the only one who at the end of the day signs the contract and takes over full responsibility. And it is only you who can accept or reject advice. Whatever you do, do your homework and don't rush into it. That's the best bit of advice anyone can give you.

Becoming a practice owner is such a big step that I think it is worthwhile repeating the main points from this section.

You should:

- never make the leap into the venture because it seems like a good idea
- never make important decisions without first talking them through with family, friends and professional advisers, and with those who have 'done it already'
- remember that some dentists (good and bad) simply are not businessmen or businesswomen and are not cut out to be business owners. Make sure you find out which category you come under *before* it's too late. Carry out a SWOT analysis on yourself
- think about the style of practice you want. Don't rush into buying the first one that comes along thinking that if you don't buy this one you'll miss the boat. If you are setting up a cold squat ask yourself, 'Why has no one set up here before?' Is it because they have looked at it and decided that it simply would not work?
- surround yourself with excellent advisers who really understand dental businesses. You want an accountant who is a member of NASDAL. Your solicitor should also be a member

of NASDAL. You want a bank manager whose clients are mostly dentists and who therefore knows the dental business

- prepare yourself for practice ownership before, not after, you own a practice
- never overstretch your finances; borrowing money might be (relatively) easy; paying it back is the hard part!
- get your accountant to work out some financial projections for you and if the figures don't stack up, walk away from the deal
- thoroughly research the market beforehand; the current owner may have survived quite happily where they are for years, but if there's another recently opened practice in the area, are you going to enjoy the same easy ride?
- have a high-quality business plan, which contains marketing and financial plans. Successful businesses all start out with a detailed, carefully worked out business plan
- listen to professional advisers; you're paying them for their expertise, so listen to what they have to say
- employ the right people
- never forget that although it may be hard to do, if at any time during the purchasing or setting up process you realise that you are making a big mistake, pull out. If you don't you will regret it in the long term.

Hold this thought: failure to research and plan does not necessarily mean that your practice will fail; it might, however, mean that it takes longer to be a success.

I bought my practice 5 years post qualification, which seemed like the right time to do it. However, I had never been involved in the management of either of the two practices I had worked in as an associate, so I had no management experience. I didn't do any of the things I have advocated you should do before buying a practice, such as:

- talk my decision over with my wife, my family or friends
- prepare a business plan
- research the market
- draw up a budget and then stick to it.

I bought it because it seemed like a good idea, which is the worst reason of all!
   If I were to do it again I would definitely follow the advice I am giving you.

Section III

People

8

Developing the core values of your practice

The core values of the practice underpin everything else that follows. Some of the information in this chapter will be repeated later when you start to think about your practice mission statement and the business planning process.

Articulating and defining the core values of your practice is a great way of motivating yourself and your team. It also clearly demonstrates to your patients that you are serious about and dedicated to delivering high-quality care. Your aim should always be to put together a winning team who all get along with one another, who are all willing to work for each other, and who are all strongly motivated by your inspired leadership. But to start off with you need to think about the core values that you are going to instil into everyone who works for you, i.e. what the practice is all about.

When you analyse your business there are several fundamental areas to think about:

1. employees
2. quality
3. patients
4. continuous improvement
5. communication.

Your employees are a crucial component in your quest for quality. You must first train then trust everyone to do the right thing right first time. However, there are riders that need to be attached to this statement. Each employee must know that they are personally responsible for their own work, and that they are part of a team, so others will be monitoring their work. You cannot possibly expect them to know what to do and how to do it unless they have been shown and told, and don't forget to write it down for them to refer to when they need reminding.

New employees should have it drummed into them that the goal of your practice is total patient satisfaction, that *everyone* is involved, that the standard of quality expected in the practice is 'no failures', and that high-quality performance will be recognised and rewarded. Periodically remind all employees of these.

A mission statement is a critical element in your strategic planning framework; it is often the first step when cultural changes are being introduced. However, a mission statement on its own does not create a sense of 'mission'; that can only come from you, the practice owner, but it should provide inspiration for your employees and be a living statement that employees can translate into objectives and goals for every aspect of the practice's operations.

The end result of your core values is your patient care. Rather than simply having a vague, nebulous concept of what your practice is trying to deliver, you should instead articulate your ideas as very well-defined core values that you and your team all share. Writing your core values down and periodically revisiting them will help you retain your focus and hence maintain the delivery of quality care for which you are striving.

Patient care programme

Patients are the life-blood of your practice, but to make a success of your business you need to be more than just a good dentist. You and your employees must show your patients that you care, over and above any legal responsibility imposed by the CQC. (More about CQC later.) You should be caring for your patients because you want to, not because you have to. Your own patient care programme should be so good that it maximises the number of patients returning to you time after time, and makes them want to recommend your practice to their friends, relatives, neighbours and work colleagues. However, patient care is not simply about meeting their expectations; it is about exceeding them. Having an excellent patient care programme means that your business is more likely to be a success.

Hold this thought: to ignore your patients is to ignore the future of your business.

Before you think about your patient care programme, try to remember some examples of good and bad customer care that you have received from companies, shops or organisations. Why was it good? Why was it bad? Then, think about how you like to be treated when you go to, say, your GP practice, or to a hospital.

With its emphasis on quality, CQC gets a whole chapter of its own later, but for now I want to start you off thinking about what is important for a patient care programme.

The key elements of a patient care programme are:

- as the practice owner you must be fully committed to the concept. It won't work if you don't believe in it. If you don't believe in it, you have to ask yourself if you're in the right job
- you and your employees must know and understand what are your patients' needs and expectations
- you and your employees must stay close to your patients and anticipate their changing needs
- you can only establish your patients' needs and expectations by talking and listening to them, whether through direct face-to-face discussion or through surveys and questionnaires
- information the patients receive from the practice, whether it is from you, the practice manager, treatment coordinator, hygienist, therapist, nurse, or receptionist, whether it is in writing or given verbally, must always be correct
- there must be a consistent approach when dealing with patients. It is no good you telling them one thing and your employees telling them something else
- it follows that there must be excellent communication between you and your employees, and with your patients. As I said earlier, at the heart of every excellently managed business is excellent communication
- you must recruit the right employees
- all employees must be trained to continuously deliver effective patient care
- service level agreements should be in place so that all tasks in relation to patient care are completed in a timely manner. Doing things when you say you are going to is an important element of patient care
- complaints must be dealt with promptly and professionally.

The concept of customer care hasn't always been around. Through much of my early years in practice I had the attitude, as did many of my colleagues, that the patient really wasn't that important. I certainly held this view through the first 10 or so years after I became a practice owner. However, two things made me change my attitude. First, I remarried; my new wife was a bank manager and is an excellent people manager. Second, I recruited a new receptionist, who was also a first class people person. I learnt a great deal about customer care from both of them.

I was not converted overnight, but I slowly began to realise that actually my patients were important. Once I realised that I was treating people, not patients, my whole attitude to customer care changed. The difference this made to my practice was tremendous. We never looked back.

I didn't get around to doing this in my practice before I retired, but I think that having some sort of patient representative group is a really good way of engaging with your customers. I am the chairman of the patient group at my GP practice; we hold regular meetings and gather opinions and views about how well or badly the practice is performing. We help the doctors carry out patient surveys and we carefully scrutinise complaints (with patient details removed, obviously) and compliments.

Communicating with patients and potential patients has never been easier through the use of social media. Nowadays everyone seems to have a Facebook page or a Twitter account, to name but two of the most popular ones, but using these for your practice comes with a warning. Under its *Guidance on using social media, 4.2.3 of Standards for the Dental Team*, the General Dental Council (GDC) makes it very clear about what you should and should not do regarding social media. The GDC's guidance is common sense; staying within the guidelines is self-evidently important. So what is the best way to make best use of social media?

- Don't saturate your page with information but be sparing with what you post; less is more.
- Control who can post on your page; if you can't control it, don't use it.
- Rather than promote your practice on your social media pages, encourage patients to tell people about how great your practice is on theirs. Self-praise is no praise.

I was not part of the social media generation until after I'd given up dental practice. However, having embraced its use, I now use it sparingly to promote my writing. I know I sometimes tire of reading post after post (repeating the same thing) from others, so I like to keep my posts to a minimum. If I was still in practice I am not sure I would use Facebook, for example, to promote my practice. I think I'd be worried about over-egging the pudding and so putting potential patients off, and I'd have concerns about security of the information I posted.

I write fiction in my spare time, and there is a saying among writers, and a bit of a rule for creating good stories, that is that you 'Show, don't tell'. In dental practice this could mean that you show your patients what a brilliant clinician you are and what a superb practice you have by what you do, and not by telling them.

Do you need a website? I would definitely say, yes.

What should you have on your website? Anything and everything that makes it very easy for patients, but more importantly potential patients, to find you, contact you, see what you have to offer and the benefits, how much it is going to cost them, and your opening hours. Make it easy for the user and don't overload them with too much information. Remember, any information you have on your website must be kept up to date, so you will have to do this yourself or delegate responsibility.

It is worth paying a professional web designer to build your website even if you think you can do it yourself via a 'build-your-own-website' website.

Think about having an application software, an 'app', for your practice; an app simply gives users a quick link to your practice website. Apps are convenient.

We all use the Internet to search for everything and anything, but certain things put me off some sites, even before I've read what they have to say, and these are: if they are difficult to read because of poor colour contrast, poor choice of font or print size, or if things keep whizzing in and out of the screen. I hate that. I also quickly lose faith if I come across any grammatical or spelling errors on a website; if they can't get that right, can they do their job right?

I use apps a lot as a short cut to my favourite websites. Why shouldn't dental practices have them?

Hold this thought: it is no use having a website if your employees don't know the services the practice has to offer, the cost and how individual services are delivered.

As well as having a website, you must also have a well-written, professionally produced brochure. Although we live in an age when it seems as if every business, and almost everyone, has their own website, people still sometimes like something tangible to read. Telling someone to look at your website does not convey the same personal message that handing them your brochure and then inviting them to ask questions has, does it?

Whether you decide to have all of the practice information online, or online and in the form of a paper brochure, or, as more and more practices seem to be doing, as a download, what you say has to be clear and, in this very busy world, very concise. The rules of good writing apply no matter what, so it is therefore a good idea to engage a professional copywriter to help you put together the words you are going to use. That does not mean, however, that you (and/or your practice manager) should not make a start on producing a rough working draft of how you want your practice information to look and the form of words you want to use. You should begin by asking the following questions:

- Who is the information aimed at? Is it aimed at existing patients, restating information that they might already know or drawing their attention to information that perhaps they weren't aware of? Or is it aimed primarily at prospective patients?
- What do you want to tell them?
- What is going to be the structure and format of the information?
- What is the budget?

The social class of the audience is largely irrelevant: educated people will expect the information to be written in good English; less well educated people need to have it spelled out in plain, easy to understand English. There might be a difference in readership between *The Times* and the red tops, but they are both well written.

Hold this thought: the average reading age of the UK population is 11 years, so if the message is not clear it will fall on deaf ears and blind eyes.

Unless your practice is limited to certain types of treatment, don't focus too closely on special interests. Don't restrict your potential market. The vast majority of people are not looking for specialists in the first instance; they just want a dentist.

What is the message going to be?

- People know that dentists do dentistry, so don't waste space telling them that the practice does fillings, root treatment, crowns and bridges etc.
- People want to know why they should come to your practice as opposed to the one down the road; spell out the benefits.
- Don't try to explain what gum disease is, what different types of bridges are made of, or why a crown might be necessary on a tooth.
- Does it really need to be pointed out that your employees have been trained and that the practice sterilises its instruments, or that it is registered with the CQC?

The phrasing of the text should reflect a confident, positive and professional tone. The text should be:

- clear: decide what the message is and say it in as few words as are necessary; avoid tautology, poor syntax and unnecessary punctuation; use familiar words because the reader is more likely to understand what is being said
- concise: avoid verbosity and technical language
- correct; is the information up to date and accurate?

The information should be set out logically in easy-to-read headed sections as bullet points. People are too busy to bother reading through long paragraphs; they want information in easy-to-read, small, easily digestible chunks.

Many of the phrases used in off-the-shelf practice websites and brochures are glib. They contain such things as 'If you are a new patient, we would like to take this opportunity to welcome you to this practice.' Anyone looking for a new dentist who collects several brochures or reads several websites bearing the same greeting will judge them all to be disingenuous. Try to come up with something original, phrases that reflect the 'feel' of your practice.

When you have finished, have your draft text checked by a professional copywriter or, if you have any English teachers among your patients, ask one of them if they would kindly read it through for you. Producing a finished brochure or ending up with a website that contain glaring errors undermines people's confidence in the organisation that produced it.

My wife and I were having lunch in a restaurant on one of the Greek islands when the owner asked if we'd mind checking his English version of his menu, the original of which was obviously in Greek. He recognised the need to present his menu to his English diners in very clear and well-written English.

I practised in the pre-online age, when practices had paper brochures. When it came to writing my practice brochure, I wanted something that was different from all the others. I wanted something that was personal to the practice and which reflected our new customer care focus.

I first found out what information I had to include; I then got hold of as many brochures as I could from other practices. I edited and re-edited, drafted and redrafted, played around with the layout, and asked my employees and family to read it and to offer suggestions about how I could improve it. The whole process took weeks, but it was worth it.

I also wrote a brochure titled *Dentistry for Children – A Parents' Guide*, which I used in my practice.

Despite there being so much information available at the press of a button, there is no substitute for old-fashioned personal contact: train your staff to communicate verbally and face to face with people.

People in business often talk about putting the customer first, when most of the time this is not what they practise. Sincerity is an important part of your patient care programme, sincerity not only from you, but also from everyone else in your team. Patients are not stupid and they will see right through a practice where everyone says 'Yes, yes, yes' when they really mean 'No, no, no.'

Hold this thought: a false smile fools no one.

After every tooth extraction, no matter how simple it was for me (an extraction is never a 'simple' procedure for a patient) I'd give the patient the usual post-operative instructions. Our care did not stop there: I or my nurse or my receptionist would phone the patient later that day and make sure that they were alright. This reassurance was very much appreciated. You can never do too much for your patients.

Your practice charter

One way in which you can set out an overview of how the practice deals with its patients and what it expects in return from them is to have a practice charter. Everyone in the practice should be involved in its production and it needs to be something you all agree on.

The charter falls into two sections: first, what the practice will do and, second, what the patients' responsibilities are to the practice.

You could list what patients can expect from the practice. For example:

- to be greeted in a friendly and welcoming manner at all times
- the practice to be clean and comfortable
- to be offered advice and information relevant to their own particular dental health problems
- confidentiality at all times
- to be referred to the appropriate specialist when necessary
- during normal opening hours, patients with problems to be seen as soon as possible
- to be seen as near to their appointment time as possible; if there is a delay they will be told
- any complaints to be treated fairly by the practice.

The list is there to give patients a 'flavour' of how the practice deals with its customers. However, it is a two-way process, and you need to also set out clearly what the patients have to do in return, namely:

- to be courteous to all members of the practice team
- to value their dental health and therefore take advice from the dentist and their employees
- to keep their appointments and be on time
- to give reasonable notice if they are unable to keep an appointment so that someone else can be seen in their place – the practice can charge for failed appointments
- to respect the need for the dentist and their employees to have adequate time off.

This charter encapsulates the 'contract' between the practice and its customers. It should be on your website.

Hold this thought: people like to know where they stand, whether it be with other people or with organisations; this is why communication is so important.

9

Managing patients

The clinical management of patients is outside the scope of this book, but leaving treatment aside, every patient has to be 'managed'.

Nor is this a psychology book. However, the Colour Code Personality Profile, created by Dr Taylor Hartman, divides people's personalities into four colours, which might prove useful to you:

- Red (the power wielders)
- Blue (the do-gooders)
- White (the peacekeepers)
- Yellow (the fun lovers).

(Hartman, Taylor. *The Color Code*, p. 40.)

Roughly speaking, Reds make up 25% of the population, Blues 35%, Whites 20%, and Yellows 20%. The same spread of personalities will be present in your patients.

What colour produces what type of patient?

Picking some of the characteristics of each colour, and tying them in with how they might present as dental patients, I think these are the things you should be on the lookout for.

Reds are the power wielders of the world. Their strengths are that they are assertive, confident and determined. They often have to be right and they tend to be poor listeners. So, even though you are the dentist, they will probably try to tell you what to do! But watch out if things go wrong because they can come across as harsh and critical, even when they don't mean to be.

Blues love commitment and they thrive on relationships. They are highly committed and loyal. However, they are highly demanding perfectionists who are mistrusting and prone to worry about nearly everything, which makes them insecure. They are also judgemental. Lacking trust, they are resentful or unforgiving. They often fail to see anything positive. They are the most controlling of the four colours.

Whites will do anything to avoid confrontation, so they are patient and accepting. They don't share what they are feeling, understanding or seeing, so you may never know if they like what you have done for them.

I had a male patient, in his mid to late fifties, who had run his own successful business, which he sold in his forties, and who then spent his time on the golf course and cruising around the world. He was always very courteous, if not a little abrupt, towards me, and we only ever used titles and surnames to address one other. To say that he was difficult to treat was an understatement. I dreaded him coming in because I knew that whatever I said he would question, and that whatever I did just did not seem to work. Anyhow, this went on for years, and I suppose he must have trusted me because he kept coming back. And then one day, a Friday afternoon, he presented as an emergency with a broken tooth. My worst nightmare! Anyhow, the tooth had to come out, and after I'd removed it, we both gave a big sigh of relief. The outcome, however, was better than I had hoped for, because this 'Red' person admitted that ever since childhood he had been terrified of the dentist and that I was the only dentist he had ever trusted. His abruptness and the reason why he had been difficult to treat were a direct consequence of his absolute fear, which, because of his personality, he had tried to hide or cover up. I now understood him. He continued to come to me for his dental care, and although he was not always easy to treat, our relationship changed so that I no longer dreaded treating him and he no longer lived in fear of the dentist.

Yellows are enthusiastic and are always looking for something new. They develop friendships with ease, but are very self-centred.

Your patient list will be made up of every type of personality. You might like treating a certain type of patient: the compliant, easy-to-please, always grateful ones, who it doesn't matter what you do or say to them, they are never going to complain. Unfortunately life is never that simple.

There is a great deal of psychology involved in dentistry, and taking time to get to know your patients and what makes them tick helps to make your and their lives a little easier.

Getting off to a flying start

If your first patient of the day is booked in for 9 a.m., it is common courtesy to see them *at* 9 a.m. and not at 9.15 a.m. – because you, your nurse or the receptionist (or all three of you) are slow at preparing to work. Patients become even more anxious if you keep them waiting.

Having the practice open and ready to see its first customer on time should be part of your customer care programme.

Pay your employees for an 'extra' half hour each day: 15 minutes before the practice officially opens and 15 minutes at the end of the day. If you pay them for 15 minutes after you are supposed to finish seeing patients they will have enough time to clear up and make a start on setting the surgery up for the next day. The receptionist has time to calmly deal with the last patient, and won't be preoccupied with catching the bus! The nurse won't be rushing off before the last patient is out of the chair, leaving the surgery in a mess, which will all have to be cleared away before you can see your first patient the following morning. Giving your employees the time each morning to check the day list, prepare the surgery and get all of the day's laboratory work out, means that you will not be playing catch-up as soon as you step through the front door. (Laboratory work should always be back at least one day, if not two, before the patient's next appointment, and you or your nurse should always check that the technician has done exactly what you asked them to do.) It also means that your receptionist can listen to any messages on the telephone answering machine without them being overheard by other patients – patient confidentially is very important.

> My nurse and I used to take an extra 5 or 10 minutes in the morning going through the day list. We'd identify any potential problems, whether it be with treatment, time keeping or simply the patient. I was determined that the day would go smoothly, without any hitches. I also used to keep an eye on the hygienist's list because some of my patients would be booked in with her as well and I didn't want to disrupt my hygienist's day because of problems in my surgery.

Managing children *and* their parents

Treating children is for many dentists a very stressful experience. Having to deal with their parents can be even more stressful. I have an MSc in Children's Dentistry, and so I naturally used to see and treat a large number of children, some of whom were registered with the practice and some who were referred to me by colleagues. The brochure I wrote and used to use in my practice, *Dentistry For Children – A Parents' Guide*, was my way of giving parents all the information I wanted them to have about how my employees and I were going to care for and treat their child(ren). Parents often commented on how useful the brochure was.

The focus of my brochure is very much about communication, communication between the dentist and the child, the parent and the child (in the context of the child's dental care), and the parent and the dentist. This 'triangle' is the key to developing a good rapport between all three parties. During all my years as a clinician I found that whenever there was a problem with communication between me and a parent, there were inevitably problems managing their child's behaviour in the surgery.

To start off with, some parents don't see their child's baby (deciduous) teeth as being important. Getting the message across that baby teeth *are* important is a good place to start.

Parents generally have little idea about when they should start to take their child to the dentist, so tell them: the earlier the better.

One of the major problems with treating children is that they often come to the dentist having already been told or having heard negative things about the dentist that fill them with dread. Counter this negative message.

If you can train the parents, you are halfway there to being able to manage their children. Setting out a very clear list of dos and don'ts, which the parents will hopefully take heed of, helps enormously.

> A girl of about 7 or 8 years of age was brought to see me by her dad. She had a history of irregular attendance at a number of other practices, and a fear and dislike of dentists. Oh, joy, I thought. At the first visit she needed a great deal of coaxing to even sit in the dental chair, but Dad sat quietly, though obviously concerned and a little embarrassed, in the chair in the corner of the surgery. I made some progress, and after discussing his daughter's treatment plan, Dad made a second appointment for her.
>
> At her next appointment, the girl went immediately to sit in the chair; I was able to carry out some simple treatment on her without any problems. Afterwards, I asked Dad (out of earshot of the girl) why she'd been so much better today. His reply was that after last time, he'd promised to buy her a pony if she behaved. Bribery worked this time, but I wonder what he'd have to buy her in future every time she didn't want to do something.

Parents want to know what will happen during their child's first visit. Assuming that a child does not require emergency treatment, then you can reassure them by telling them what will happen.

Cooperation between you, the parent and the child is important if the goals of the child's dental care are to be achieved. It is important that a relationship of mutual trust and understanding develops between all three parties. An initially difficult child will gain confidence and develop the trust needed to become calm, unafraid and cooperative when the parent and dentist work together. Reinforce this message by telling the parent that by all working together a positive attitude in the child can develop, which leads to a lifetime of good dental experiences. This communication triangle (child, parent and dentist) is a very important part of a child's long-term dental care.

Parents naturally worry about what is going to happen if you ever have to carry out treatment on their child. To help allay their fears, tell the parent that once their child has been examined and you have discussed any proposed treatment with them, a treatment plan will be drawn up. You should add that children are introduced to dentistry gently, usually by having a simple procedure carried out at the first visit (tell, show and do is a good approach to adopt) and that pain control is used whenever it is clinically necessary.

Parents in the surgery is a divisive issue, not only between parents and dentists, but between dentists themselves. What do you think? Maybe it's best to sit on the fence and tell parents that the practice has no hard-and-fast rules about whether parents are allowed into, or are excluded from, the surgery. You can tell them that some children react well when a parent is present in the surgery and others behave better when their parent remains in reception.

Parents often believe that if they are excluded from the surgery they are abandoning their child. It is important that you reassure them by saying that sometimes their presence can undermine communication and rapport between you (the dentist) and the child, and the only way to regain the child's attention is by the parent being elsewhere. You should decide, based on your experience and knowledge, whether it is in the child's best interest to have their parent in the treatment room. In my experience, an uncooperative child will almost always calm down and cooperate if the parent is out of sight.

> Nothing I ever did in dentistry gave me more professional satisfaction than seeing a child progress from an anxious individual to a dentally confident patient, and usually with a caries- and restoration-free adult dentition. This never happened unless I had established great communication with the child *and* with their parent(s) or guardian from the outset.

Don't forget to also dish out loads of dental health advice to parent and child.

You and your team should all undertake some form of training in how to successfully manage and care for this vulnerable group.

Hold this thought: every child you treat must be managed in accordance with CQC standards.

Managing the elderly

Managing elderly patients presents its own challenges. Reduced mobility means they take longer to walk from the waiting room to your surgery, so perhaps you need to think about allowing more time for their appointments. Perhaps you have to start seeing them in a downstairs surgery and not in the one upstairs? Deterioration in their general health and perhaps increased and constantly changing medication means you have to be more diligent in your medical history taking. A worsening memory or general mental capacity means you will have to spend more time explaining things to them and making sure they understand everything that is said or presented to them. Hearing problems can compromise your ability to communicate effectively with them. Perhaps they start to forget their appointments.

The UK's population is ageing and so you cannot ignore this ever-growing group.

You and your team should all undertake some form of training in how to successfully manage and care for this vulnerable group.

> If you've ever worked in the same practice for a number of years you will have seen how your patients age. This is of course part of a natural cycle, but it also means that in some cases you have to change or modify the way you treat someone, which I know I had to do during my 25 years in one practice.

Hold this thought: every elderly person you treat must be managed in accordance with CQC standards.

Managing people with special needs

Patients of all ages with special needs require special care and understanding from everyone at the practice. Your team should have a good working knowledge of mental and physical impairment issues, and should all know how to communicate and interact with such patients in an understanding and compassionate way.

You might want to consider having an access statement that describes the practice's facilities and services for people with access difficulties, and to ensure that it is available to prospective patients.

An access statement should be part of your customer care programme. An access statement is a description of your facilities and services to inform people with access needs. All areas of the practice should be described.

You and your team should all undertake some form of training in how to successfully manage and care for this vulnerable group.

Children, the elderly and patients of all ages with special needs require more time and a great deal of patience from you and your team.

> I once worked in a practice where the principal used nitrous oxide on *every* child he treated, irrespective of whether or not they had any behavioural or management issues. He obviously saw this as a quick and easy way of completing the treatment, but with little regard for the child's long-term wellbeing.

Hold this thought: every patient with special needs, and those who are vulnerable, must be managed in accordance with CQC standards.

Managing domiciliary visits

Whether you regard domiciliary visits as a chore or part of the service you provide, you should make sure that they are well managed and cost effective.

Decide from the outset what type of treatments you are happy to carry out in a domestic setting. Some dentists limit the treatments to scalings, simple fillings (without the use of a motorised drill), simple extractions, and dentures. You could go as far as investing in a portable and domiciliary dental unit so that you are able to offer a wider range of treatments. Whichever of these options you choose, you should:

- brief your receptionist so they know how long you need for any particular appointment, which will depend on the location of the visit, and the physical and mental health of the patient
- put together a domiciliary kit (use a plastic crate with a fitted lid); this is best done by your nurse, but then checked by you
- discuss with your nurse beforehand any modifications you might make to your normal clinical routines, for example, moisture control when carrying out a simple filling
- make sure that your receptionist contacts the patient *before* you leave the practice so that you know that the patient is at home. Unplanned, emergency or urgent doctor or hospital appointments by the patient could mean you make a wasted journey
- ensure that after every domiciliary visit your nurse cleans and sterilises the things you used, and that the domiciliary kit is restocked.

One thing you should bear in mind when offering domiciliary visits, especially where dentures are concerned, is that if you are going to ease or adjust dentures you will either have to have a portable drill or be prepared to collect the denture, ease it in your surgery, then return it to the patient, usually at no charge. This can quickly eat into your profit.

If you really don't want to do domiciliary visits or, if you are contacted by a patient who needs, for example, more complex dental care, consider referring them to a mobile dental service, or to a nearby colleague who is able to carry out the treatment.

> I used to block book domiciliary; that way they didn't disrupt the smooth running of a normal day in the surgery too much. However, it used to annoy me when my nurse and I would turn up at a nursing home for a pre-booked appointment, only to find they weren't ready for us! I quickly learnt to phone the nursing home first.

Hold this thought: every patient you treat in a domiciliary setting must be managed in accordance with CQC standards.

Managing your 'new' patients

As Section II was all about buying your first practice, I thought it would be useful to say something about what you should do if your 'new' patients need a great deal of treatment, that is, if their previous dentist hasn't looked after them. How do you manage what can be a stressful situation for any dentist, let alone a new practice owner?

Taking over a new practice full of (new) patients can be problematic. You may experience resistance, especially if you are a young dentist taking over from an older colleague, to new treatments, or even to treatment itself. Don't take this resistance personally: be prepared to answer questions (lots of them) and be prepared for people saying 'No'. You never know, having thought about it, they might one day return, happy to have you do the treatment. Managing what is commonly known as supervised neglect is tricky and can be very unnerving for the young, conscientious practitioner. Here is a strategy that I hope will help you if and when you ever have to deal with a patient whose previous dental care has been substandard, and who is now under your care.

Fresh out of dental school, you may have been all too ready to criticise another dentist's work because, in your opinion, it is not textbook standard. As you grow longer in the tooth you come to realise that this is not always a good way to conduct yourself. However, situations may arise when you have to nail your colours to the mast and say to a patient that the work they have just paid a great deal of money for is, well, frankly, not very good, or that their previously undiagnosed periodontal disease really does need treating. You should, however, always bear in mind that we live in an increasingly litigious society and that there are people out there who don't need any encouragement to engage a solicitor to pursue a claim for compensation. Take care that you aren't unwittingly sucked into this by being too critical of a colleague's work.

No one has a problem with the correct treatment being done well. Problems start to creep in when the correct treatment is done badly. Sometimes the wrong treatment is done, though sometimes well. Even worse, though, is when the wrong treatment is done badly. I suppose the worst situation is when treatment is not done at all – so-called supervised neglect.

> When I became a practice owner I knew that I would (hopefully) be seeing many of my patients for years to come. The danger, as I saw it, was falling into the trap of not looking closely enough. To prevent this happening I resolved from day one to regard every patient I saw and every mouth I examined as if it was the first time I'd ever seen that person or that mouth. This strategy served me well over 20-plus years.

You will have your own clinical standards, which will have evolved from your undergraduate days, which were then influenced by other dentists with whom you worked, and also by any formal or informal training you have undertaken since you graduated. If you are going to criticise another dentist's work, you need to start thinking like an expert witness and know something about clinical negligence law.

But by what standards does the law judge clinical dentistry? At the time of writing there are two legal tests that a dental expert witness must apply when giving their opinion. The law imposes a duty of care on clinicians; it expects them to always act in a reasonable, responsible and respectable way towards the patients in their care. However, this approach was criticised because it meant that if the accused dentist could find an expert who would testify that they would have done the same thing, that was a defence. This legal test was modified so that the professional opinion that may be called upon to support a defence has to be capable of withstanding logical analysis. Looking at things from your perspective, you should always make sure that the treatment, care and advice you give to your patients can be defended as being logical.

The word the law uses to describe poor or bad dentistry is 'substandard'. Hence, when you are assessing someone else's work that you think is substandard, you have to ask yourself two questions, which are, 'How would a reasonable, responsible and respectable body of dental practitioners have conducted themselves?' and 'Can I provide a logical explanation for what was actually done (or omitted) knowing all of the facts of the case?' These questions throw up some key points for you to think about: 'dental practitioners', i.e. *not* specialist endodontist, periodontist etc., or hospital-based consultants. If the treatment was carried out in general practice by a general practitioner, that's the standard you should apply and the one that the courts will also apply. Then there's the point about 'knowing all the facts of the case', which if you are going to rely solely on what the patient tells you and what you have found during your examination, might not be 'all of the facts'. You must remember that the treatment or lack of treatment must be seen in context. How often have you not been able to do as good a job as you had wished simply because the patient was very difficult to work on? Would another dentist, on viewing your handiwork, say that it was substandard? Anything that has prevented you from doing your job well should be noted in the patient records, for example: 'Patient very fidgety',

'Patient refused more local despite telling me they could feel it when I was preparing cavity'. Patients who present with apparently untreated, long-standing periodontal disease, for example, may have been attending their dentist for years and have been ignoring their advice. But they aren't always going to tell you that, are they? Patients are not passive receivers of treatment, care or advice, so be wary about taking their side of the story at face value, at least not until you have *all* of the facts.

If you are confronted with a patient who you think has received substandard treatment and/or care, what should you do? I would not voice any opinion until I was in possession of the full facts of the case. The patient may know that things are not right and will probably ask you what you think. Bat their questions aside for now, saying that you need more information and that you need more time to think about his or her case. You should ask them to come back so that you can conduct a more extensive assessment and investigation (I would always do this for free). It is crucial that you gather as much information as you can. You must always ensure that your records would stand up to the closest scrutiny.

Your discussions with the patient need to be as non-committal as you can make them, with nothing coming from you that could be construed as encouraging them to pursue a claim for clinical negligence. If they ask you whether you think the treatment or care they have had is poor, again you must make it clear that although you have examined them, you were not present when the treatment or care was given and so are unable to say for certain one way or the other. They may ask that if they do go to a solicitor, would you support their case. Again, you must remain professional and say that if that happened you would of course be prepared to let the solicitor have all of your records to assist you with the case. Remember that you might one day have to stand up in court and defend what you have said. One thing that an expert witness is not is a judge, and you must not put yourself into that role. If you are unsure about a particular case, you should always consult your defence organisation from the outset.

I'm not saying that you should always turn a blind eye to substandard treatment, or that you should not carry out your duty of care to your patients by not being open and upfront about their current dental health. However, experience teaches that not everyone or everything is perfect, and that sometimes you have to accept that. My advice is to be pragmatic rather than dogmatic, and not to be too judgemental.

Hold this thought: communication is not only the secret of a successful business, it is also at the heart of patient management.

Section 1 introduced you to the principles of management, so it might help if you relate what you do with your patients to what you are going to have to do in terms of managing your practice. With a patient, you first have to:

- take and record their medical history
- take and record their dental history
- take and record their social history
- carry out a comprehensive extra-oral and intra-oral examination
- perhaps you have to carry out special tests
- arrive at a diagnosis
- formulate a short-, medium- and long-term treatment plan.

(Your treatment plan should always be about solving a patient's needs.)

This is the information-gathering phase of the 'Planning' part of the management cycle.

Once you have planned the patient's treatment, you have to specify the appointments they are going to need (not just how long each appointment should be, but when they should be), make sure that you'll have a nurse to assist you, and that the equipment and materials you are going to need will all be on hand. The receptionist books the appointments. You finally carry out the treatment. You should then review the outcome of the treatment, which might make you change how you would do similar treatment in the future. In all, this is the planning, organising, implementing and control or review of the management cycle.

Central to the management of all of your patients is the management of your appointment book, i.e. management of your time. Making the best use of your time so that you maximise your income, while at the same time ensuring that you do not overrun and are not, therefore, constantly keeping patients waiting, is something you must quickly learn how to do.

The essence of time management is the division of a piece of work into a series of component parts or stages. This might be relatively easy to do. However, have you ever analysed how you spend your time each day? How efficient is your time management? Could you reduce the time you allocate to, say, an examination on a regular attender with a very well maintained mouth, without compromising the standard of your history taking or the clinical examination? Do all the 5 minutes you have left at the end of every 30-minute appointment add up to being able to see one more patient per day? Adopting efficient working habits is something you should do while you have the luxury of time. Making yourself and those around you be more efficient when you have, for example, financial pressures is a lot more difficult.

When thinking about how to work more efficiently begin with the idea that your practice needs to run like an extremely efficient engine. Every cog must be in the right place at the right time and running in harmony at the correct speed if the engine is to be effective. An engine is not working properly if much of the energy you put into it is dissipated or lost within the engine before it is put to use. Think about how you get the right cogs in the right place and all moving in harmony at the correct speed. Have you even got the right number of cogs?

Your appointment book is the key to your time management. Factor in not only how long it is going to take you to physically do the treatment, but also for such things as whether the patient likes to talk a lot before they sit in the chair, whether injections tend to take longer to work, or whether the patient is just downright awkward.

A number of years ago I was involved with a practice that had just moved from the NHS to a private practice. Instead of the quick 5 or 10-minute check-ups, the principal thought they would now have the luxury of taking half an hour. The first thing to say is that their charge for these two check-ups in an hour equated to not much more they were earning under the old system; second, check-ups under the new system were only taking them 20 minutes to complete so in every hour they were sitting around for a third of the time. Their hourly rate had in fact fallen. Solution? Cut the appointment time down to 20 minutes and see three patients in an hour. Result? Fifty per cent increase in income.

Managing emergency appointments

Managing emergencies without letting them disrupt the smooth running of your appointment book is never easy. There are, however, a number of ways in which you can try to manage emergency appointments.

- Leave it to chance, hoping that a patient will cancel at short notice or fail to attend, leaving a gap in the book.
- Set aside dedicated 'Emergency' slots, which are not to be used for anything other than emergencies.
- Use the end of the morning or afternoon sessions to see them.

One of the most distressing emergencies in general practice is the child who has had an accident and who has damaged their teeth. This child should whenever possible be seen and be seen immediately, which means that your clinical team has to know how to deal with this situation effectively and efficiently so that it does not disrupt the smooth running of the practice any more than it has to. Training is the key.

You should experiment with various emergency booking arrangements until you find one that works for you. However, should you change your system, make sure that every one of your staff knows about it.

Over the years I tried all sorts of ways of fitting emergencies into what were usually already very busy days. Find a system that works for you (your employees might not like working through their lunch hour or staying late after work). Discuss in your team meetings how emergencies can best be handled.

Managing failed appointments

This is a tricky topic and one about which I am not sure anyone has the definitive answer, but I'll try to give some tips on how to reduce it, if not eliminating it entirely.

Failed appointments, or 'DNAs', cost your business money; every lost hour of work is probably losing you hundreds of pounds of income, income you can never recover.

Why do people DNA? Forgetfulness, laziness, something better turned up, a lack of respect for you as a professional, are just some of the reasons, I suspect. Unless you are so desperate to hang on to every patient, get rid of persistent offenders. Write to them telling them to go somewhere else and enclose a bill for all of your time they've wasted.

One of the big problem with managing DNAs is that occasionally receptionists forget to record in the notes that the patient phoned the practice the day before to cancel their appointment. A DNA letter is therefore sent, the patient complains and the practice loses what was a conscientious patient. Practice records *must* be very accurate if you are going to start charging every patient who DNAs.

One thing I have heard of that one dentist does to manage DNAs is to send out a standard letter, but to then hand-write on it something along the lines that they won't charge this time, but will in future. This makes the dentist seem like a reasonable person, while at the same time chastising the patient but leaving the door open for them to return. Don't be so generous with repeat offenders.

Trying to identify likely offenders is not all that easy, but as you should do when monitoring and hopefully controlling employee absenteeism, so you should record all DNAs. You will find that 80% of your DNAs are down to 20% of your patients – this is known as the Pareto principle. Identify the 20% who are responsible, deal with them, and 80% of your DNAs will disappear overnight.

Many organisations use texts to remind their customers about their appointment. This is a low-cost option and is something you should do.

When should you refer a patient?

There are, as far as I am aware, no hard and fast rules about when a dentist should refer a patient for specialist treatment, nor are there any guidelines issued by the GDC, other than the maxim 'Put patients' interests first'. In this context, if you ever have the misfortune to be called before the GDC they will want to establish whether you were sufficiently qualified and competent to provide the treatment which you proposed for that patient, and whether or not it was in the patient's best interest. You should always be prepared and willing to refer any patient whose treatment is beyond you. There are, however, other factors to take into account when considering making referral.

I suppose the best advice is to ask yourself the following questions:

- Am I competent to provide the treatment I know this patient needs?
- Is the patient making demands upon my clinical judgement and pushing me to provide treatment that I am not sure is in their best interests?
- Am I able to solve this patient's problems?
- When something has gone wrong, am I capable of putting it right?
- Are the patient and I getting on? Do they trust my advice and my judgement?

Some dentists will not admit to patients or to themselves that there is some dentistry that they are not capable of doing to an adequate standard. Rather than admit this, they press on and invariably end up with problems. In my opinion, it is a good dentist who knows his or her limitations and is willing to refer a patient rather than attempt the treatment him- or herself.

Some patients can be demanding: they read about dental techniques in the lay press and on the Internet, and come in almost telling you to do such and such a treatment. These 'Internet dentists' are not worth the effort. Don't fall into the trap of trying to please this type of patient.

There will be times when despite your best effort you are unable to solve a patient's problems, whether it be the alleviation of pain or a tricky aesthetic problem. Don't persevere; send them to someone who is better qualified.

When things go wrong (as they sometimes do), if you think you are unable to put things right or if you feel out of your depth, again, send them on to someone with more experience and knowledge.

Rapport is important and if you feel, for whatever reason, that you and the patient are not seeing eye to eye, call it a day and send them to someone else.

How you make the referral is important. Don't leave the note telling you to do the referral sitting on your desk for weeks, not even for days; do it today. Do you use email or send a hard copy letter in the post? Emails are not always secure so unless you've gone to the trouble and the expense of encrypting all emails that are sent from your practice, don't use email.

The letter you send and the way in which you ask a colleague to temporarily take over responsibility for the care and treatment of your patient must be done on a professional basis. First, the letter.

- Use the name, title and job title of the person to whom you are referring the patient.
- If you are referring to a department in a hospital, address the letter to the head of that department.
- Provide full details about the patient you are referring: their full name, title, date of birth, and contact details.
- Give a short, but yet detailed summary of why you are referring the patient.
- Include any relevant x-rays etc. and any relevant correspondence.
- Indicate what outcome you expect from the referral.

Don't forget to use the correct form of salutation and to sign the letter off in the correct manner. If you know the name of the person to whom you are writing, address them as 'Dear Mr Smith' or 'Dear Mrs Jones', or 'Dear Ms Black' if you aren't sure of a woman's marital status. Sign the letter off with 'Yours sincerely'. If you don't know the name of the person to whom you are writing, address him or her as 'Sir' or 'Madam', or, if you are not sure of the person's gender, address him or her as 'Sir/Madam, or 'Sir or Madam'. Sign this letter off with 'Yours faithfully'. All of this is simply good professional etiquette.

> At one time I worked in the Admissions Department of a dental hospital, and you would not believe the number of patients we used to see whose dentist had sent them in with a referral letter that simply said 'Please see and treat.' These dentists hadn't even taken the time to write a decent referral, and in some cases the poor patient didn't even know why they'd been sent to us. It was as if the dentist just wanted to get the patient off their hands and pass them on to someone else to deal with. At least the dentist had said 'Please'!

You should ask the patient if they would like to have a copy of the referral letter.

Hold this thought: however well or badly you treat or manage your patients, you end up with the patients you deserve.

Accepting referrals as a specialist practitioner

How do you want your colleagues to refer patients to you? There are a number of options:
- telephone
- email

- online
- letter.

You should always insist on having a paper record of any referral, so if the initial referral is made over the telephone (to expedite the process) always ask the referring practitioner to follow this up with a written request.

Email, although a written request, is not ideal because most emails are not secure.

Some practices that accept referral have an online service, usually a form that the referring practitioner fills in and then submits. I wonder if there is sufficient room on some of these forms to include a full account of the reason(s) for the referral, and there is often no place for a signature.

A letter is the best way to refer. It provides a permanent record (important for medico-legal reasons) and leaves the writer free to say as much as they want about the patient and their problems.

It is tempting to try to make the referral process as simple and straightforward as possible to help any dentist who wants to send a patient to you. By all means keep the process simple, but don't cut corners when it comes to the exchange of information or communication between you and the other dentist/practice. Decide what information you would like to have and then make sure everyone knows; that way you make your life as simple as it can be. You should always ask for and expect to have:

- the name and title (if appropriate) of the person who has referred the patient
- full details about the patient being referred: their full name, title, date of birth, and contact details. (It is a good idea to also ask how the patient would like to be contacted and, if by telephone, when is the best time.)
- a detailed summary of why the patient has been referred
- relevant x-rays etc. and any relevant correspondence
- an indication of the outcome the referring dentist expects from the referral.

This is the other side of the coin to what was said a few pages earlier, except that it is presented from the specialist's perspective.

Once you have received the request to see a patient, it is up to you to make sure that the process of booking them in runs as smoothly as possible.

- Your receptionist should contact them within a day or two of receipt of the referral. (You may choose to contact the patient yourself.)
- It should always be made very clear who is contacting the patient and why.
- The initial appointment is made, and if this is done over the telephone, written confirmation should be sent by first-class post by way of confirmation.
- The receptionist should ask the patient if they have any questions and should answer these as fully as possible.
- The patient should be given information about directions to the practice, parking facilities etc. Nothing should be left to chance.

Hold this thought: the personal touch is a very important part of running a specialist, referral-based practice.

Managing patient complaints: turning complaints into compliments

No matter how well you think you are caring for your patients you are likely at some time to get complaints. Whatever the current protocols are for handling complaints under the NHS, or those from private patients under the Dental Complaints Service, it is good practice to have your own very robust complaints policy and procedure.

What is a complaint? Basically it is an expression of dissatisfaction that requires a response. What do patients complain about? Basically, anything and everything. They will complain about:

- treatment

- service: cost, pain (continuing, or being ignored), conduct (including rudeness), getting access or not getting access to treatment, giving or not giving consent
- communication: lack of it is usually at the heart of most complaints. Most complaints are about dentists, but some are about other members of the dental team.

What are people looking for when they make a complaint? It might simply be an apology. There is anecdotal evidence that some complaints escalate because someone did not say 'Sorry' at the outset. An apology is not an admission of liability or guilt, so don't feel that you should never apologise.

People often want an explanation and want to know:

- What happened?
- Why did it happen?
- What will be done to put things right?
- What action will be taken to resolve the matter?
- What is being done to stop this happening again?

You have an ethical duty and an obligation to address any complaint, no matter how unfounded you think it may be. Notwithstanding these obligations, your practice complaints procedure must be rigorous, transparent and fair.

What should you do when a patient makes a complaint? The first thing you must *not* do is treat it as if it is trivial and therefore not important. Your natural reaction might be one of anger and disbelief, but you must curb your feelings and remain objective. You might decide to categorise complaints as being either 'minor' or 'major', but I think that this can be misleading and potentially confusing. It is better to regard all complaints as serious.

I heard of a dentist who had so little regard for their patients that whenever they received a letter of complaint they used to throw it in the bin. I am not sure what happened to this particular practitioner, but this sort of behaviour is unacceptable.

If the complaint is initially made verbally, ask to have it in writing (you need a permanent record for your file). If it is not clear exactly what the complaint is about ask for clarification. You do not, after all, want to resolve the wrong complaint. You should always set out to try to resolve complaints within the practice, i.e. achieve local resolution.

Acknowledge receipt of the complaint in writing. You should state your interpretation of the complaint (this will preclude possible misunderstandings later), what you are going to do next and when they can expect to hear from you again. Your initial 'holding letter' should be sent as soon as

---

Your letter acknowledging the complaint need be no more than this.

(insert the patient's name, address, and the date of your letter)

Dear (insert name of person making the complaint)

I acknowledge receipt of your letter of complaint dated (insert date).
    My understanding is that (insert outline of complaint). If this is not correct please contact (name of person and their contact details) as soon as possible.
    I am currently investigating the circumstances surrounding your complaint and you will hear from me again no later than (insert date).
    Thank you for letting me know of your concerns, and for your patience while I explore this matter fully.
    If you have any questions concerning this letter, or would like to discuss the complaint further, please contact (name of person and their contact details).

Yours sincerely

(insert name and job title).

---

possible and certainly within no more than 5 working days. Tell them that you will respond fully in no more than 10 working days. However, if you feel that you will need longer then ask if they would mind if you extended this period. Always set time limits and stick to them. Nothing will infuriate the complainant more if you don't.

The next step is to investigate the complaint and to gather all relevant information. Do not conduct a witch-hunt or pre-judge.

Hold this thought: it is a sad fact that in any given event there are always three sides to the story: yours, theirs, and somewhere in between, the truth.

You must not be selective with your evidence gathering. Keep meticulous notes of all conversations you have with other practice members about the complaint.

Once you have completed your fact-find you can either report to the patient in writing or, and this should always be your preferred option, at a face-to-face meeting. It is best to have, say, your practice manager or senior receptionist present to take notes. Suggest to the patient that they bring along a relative or a friend for support. This meeting could be crucial to the outcome of the complaint so it is important that you show the complainant that you are sympathetic to their point of view.

Hold this thought: the art of complaint resolution is conciliation, not conflict.

It is at this stage that you have the opportunity to show them that you are totally professional, reasonable and unbiased, which hopefully will impress them, and this then may greatly influence their opinion of you in the future. Conducting yourself well at this stage could not only help to (re-) build their trust in you as a dentist, but could also win their respect for you as a person.

End the meeting by agreeing what is going to be the next step. This may be the end of the matter or you may have to give an undertaking to change certain aspects of your practice's procedures so that the same thing does not happen again. You may choose to report any changes you make back to them. You may even want to thank them for drawing any shortcomings to your attention. Confirm in writing the main points of the discussion and any action points that arise.

Hold this thought: when responding to a complaint you must always address every point raised by the complainant.

The objectives of your practice-based complaints handling system should be:

- to enable your patients to express comments, suggestions and complaints to the practice whenever they feel dissatisfied with the service they have received
- to provide them with an explanation of what has happened and, where appropriate, an apology and an assurance that the practice has taken steps to prevent the problem recurring.

You can only successfully defend a complaint if you have comprehensive, contemporaneous records to support your case, and these begin with the patient records. A patient's notes or records should always contain comprehensive details about:

- their personal details
- their full, updated medical history
- a full dental history
- a social history
- any current dental complaints
- treatment plans and the likely cost
- their consent to any treatment
- what treatment they have received and why
- the type, quantity and location of any local analgesia, general anaesthesia or sedation used
- what treatment they have refused and why
- any advice they have been given
- whether or not they accepted the advice
- information about any referrals

- details of any unusual discussions or conversations, not just between the clinicians and the patient, but also between the patient and employees
- financial transactions.

Entries should be made in such a way that any employee reading the records would be able to see instantly what treatment the patient has had done, what is to be done next and why. Your nurse and receptionist should be authorised to make entries in the records when they think it is appropriate, and they should get into the habit of doing so, having first been told that anything they do write can at any time be read by the patient. Sometimes patients will say things to them that they would never say to you.

Poor records will make it more difficult for you to fight off a complaint. Excellent records won't guarantee you'll win, but they will make it less likely you'll lose. There is one message that constantly and consistently comes from the defence organisations, which is 'Keep good records!' It seems so obvious and yet some dentists refuse to heed their advice.

The majority of patient records are nowadays computerised, which may seem convenient, but it brings its own risks as far as litigation goes. The people who produce the computer programs that allow dentists to hit one key and enter 'Scale and polish' in the patient's records, or hit another key and 'Local, prep, imps, shade' miraculously appear, again, in the patient's records, have no idea about how to write good records. You need to have absolute control over what you write, total flexibility, plus the ability to vary the narrative according to circumstances.

> The first thing clinical negligence lawyers and their expert witnesses will home in on are poor clinical records when advising their client in a civil case. Computer-generated records that are no more than a scant account, which are unclear, or which are barely comprehensible are the claimant's best friend.
>
> Entries such as 'Exam. Scale and polish' say nothing about whether an examination was carried out or whether it was proposed, and the same goes for the scale and polish. It is better to write too much than too little.

Hold this thought: no records, no defence.

If despite your best efforts to resolve their complaint, the patient ends up leaving the practice, try to identify where you might have gone wrong. Sadly, it might be that the patient was never going to be satisfied with anything you did. If, however, they decide to remain at the practice, make sure that your attitude towards them does not subtly change, and that there is no animosity, such that they no longer feel welcome. The fact that they have chosen to stay says a great deal about you and your practice.

Handling complaints can sometimes be extremely difficult and is always extremely stressful; this is why you must have a good system. Everyone in your team should be familiar with and understand how the system works.

> In all the years I was in practice I was fortunate never to have a complaint against my practice or me. I maintained all the records I needed for audit and conscientiously sent them off each year to the primary care trust, but my practice-based complaints system was never 'tested', and I was curious to see whether or not it would actually work if someone did make a complaint.
>
> Together with my practice manager, we identified a patient, someone who had been with the practice for years, whom we knew was not totally happy with her new lower full denture. She had been back a few times saying that it rubbed her, but the feeling we had was that she just did not like the denture. We contacted her and encouraged her to make a formal written 'complaint'. We then went through the practice's complaints procedure to see if it worked. It did! The lady got a new denture that she was much happier with. I found out that my complaints system would work if it were ever put to the test.
>
> I did have to ask a few patients to leave the practice. I always did this in writing. I simply told them that it had become obvious that my practice was no longer able to meet their expectations. Life's too short to bother with people who you will never please.

There is always an expectation on the part of the complainant that something will be done to prevent the same thing from happening again, so see that it doesn't.

The dentist–patient relationship is not all one-way traffic: don't feel that you can never ask a patient to leave your practice. Don't make your job more difficult than it already is by continuing to deal with people you may never be able to please.

Legitimate complaints identify weaknesses in practice procedures and gaps in staff training. Very serious complaints concerning possibly sensitive professional issues should remain confidential. Less serious ones should be discussed in staff meetings and used as a way of improving the practice. How to handle complaints effectively and efficiently should be part of your customer care programme and every member of your team should receive training in how to identify and diffuse potential complaints.

How can you turn a complaint into a compliment? By dealing with it professionally, quickly putting things right and making sure that the same thing never happens again.

> I've notice a trend among companies to use the word 'feedback' when describing what is obviously a complaint from a customer. They do this because they don't have to go to all the time, trouble and expense of dealing with and responding to a 'complaint'. All expressions of dissatisfaction are complaints and require a response.

It is an unwritten law that when something goes wrong with one person, things continue to go wrong with that same person. When a business makes one mistake for a customer, they continue making mistakes, compounding the original error. However, smart businesses have latched on to the idea that if, after the first mistake, they can recover the situation and impress the customer by putting things right quickly and without anything else going wrong, the customer will be so impressed that instead of never dealing with the company again, they become converts.

Why the Data Protection Act is important

Once you start keeping information about people you are legally obliged to register with the Information Commissioner's Office (ICO) as a data controller under the Data Protection Act (DPA) 1998 (and subsequent amendments). The DPA covers the whole of the UK, unlike the Freedom of Information Act, with which it is sometimes confused, that has separate English and Welsh, and Scottish legislation.

> I have come across a few practices that profess to be registered under the Freedom of Information Act. This Act only covers a public 'right of access' to information held by public authorities.

The DPA has eight principles, which make sure that personal information is:

- fairly and lawfully processed
- processed for limited purposes
- adequate, relevant and not excessive
- accurate and up to date
- not kept for longer than necessary
- processed in line with the rights of the person whose data it is
- secure
- not transferred to other countries without adequate protection. This rules out the use of cloud-based storage, where the server is perhaps outside the UK and where governments have the right of access to the information held within.

You must always remember that when you write anything about an individual they have the right to see what you have written. If your staff are writing things in patient records, they must be made aware of this.

There was an orthodontist at the dental school where I did my undergraduate training who used to write little acronyms on his patients' record cards. 'KTBO' meant 'Kick the bugger out!' and 'BAM' meant 'Bloody awful mother!' Such comments should never be written anywhere on your patient notes. Think it, but never write it!

The DPA does not guarantee personal privacy at all costs; it aims to strike a balance between an individual's rights and the interests of those with a legitimate reason for using personal information.

How do you ensure that you comply with the DPA? Ask yourself the following questions:

- Do I really need this information?
- Do I know what I'm using it for?
- Do the people whose information I hold know that I've got it?
- Are they likely to understand what it will be used for?
- If I pass on the information would the people about whom I hold information expect me to do this?
- Is the information secure?
- Is access to information restricted only to those who need to know?
- Is the information accurate and up to date?
- Is information destroyed or deleted as soon as I have no more need for it?
- Do my employees know their duties and responsibilities under the DPA?

Managing a data subject access request

Anyone has the right under the DPA to request a copy of any information you hold about them on computer and in some manual filing systems. This is called a data subject access.

They are also entitled to be:

- given a description of the information
- told what you might use it for
- told whom you might pass it on to
- told the source(s) of the information.

You don't have to treat every request for information as a data subject access request. As a general rule it is best to treat all written requests as being data subject access requests under the DPA.

You currently have 40 days to respond to a data subject access request after you get all the information you need from the person making the request (for example, you may need to confirm that they are who they say they are). You are as well contacting your defence organisation for advice if you receive a data subject access request.

Whenever I telephone my optician (a well-known national company) to arrange an appointment, the person answering the phone naturally asks me for my name. However, before I can give them any additional information, they reel off a list of addresses of their other clients who all share the same surname as me until they get to mine. This is a breach of the DPA. Your employees must never give out information; they should always ask for it.

Further information about the DPA can be obtained from the ICO.

You should be familiar with the Access to Medical Records Act, which gives patients the right to access health information about themselves, but which seems to have been largely replaced by the DPA. Patients can ask you to see their records informally.

The DPA is just one example of the plethora of legislation, rules and regulations within which dental practices have to work. Keeping up with all this is not easy. Organisations such as the Association of Dental Managers and Administrators (ADAM) provide an information service and advice to their members, so it is worthwhile joining them. Let them do the spadework for you!

10

Managing employees

Happy families are all alike.

Every unhappy family is unhappy in its own way.

(Leo Tolstoy, *Anna Karenina***)**

This chapter is about managing *everyone* who works in your practice, and some who work outside the practice, irrespective of their contractual or legal status. I have used the term 'employee' for convenience.

A dental practice is like a family, with its own peculiar habits and ways, but I am willing to bet that the happy 'families' are the practices that are well managed, and that the unhappy ones are the ones that aren't. Your experience of the 'family' before you created your own (bought your first practice) was hopefully a happy one. However, now you have your own 'family', one in which everyone plays by your rules.

Leadership

There are hundreds, if not thousands, of sayings about leaders and leadership: here is a very small sample.

You manage things; you lead people.

(Rear Admiral Grace Murray Hopper)

Outstanding leaders go out of their way to boost the self-esteem of their personnel. If people believe in themselves it's amazing what they can accomplish.

(Sam Walton)

Leaders think and talk about the solutions. Followers think and talk about the problems.

(Brian Tracy)

There are three essentials to leadership: humility, clarity and courage.

(Fuchan Yuan)

Practice owners (and by proxy, practice managers) have to be leaders.

What is a 'leader'? Someone who directs a group of people, perhaps? Someone who is the most successful in his or her group?

Over the years there have been many theories about what makes a great leader.

- The Great Man Theory – great leaders are born, they are not made.
- The Trait Theory – great leaders possess certain common traits.
- The Behavioural Theory that focused on how leaders behaved rather than their traits.
- Those who study these things have postulated that leaders performed in certain situations or environments; take them out of these and they stop being leaders.
- More recently it has been recognised that there is often an exchange of benefits between leaders and their followers, and that the environment in which they all operate is one of mutual positive reinforcement. People work better when their good points are valued rather than the focus always being on their bad points.

Hold this thought: excellent leaders value those around them.

How do you become or make yourself a great leader? First, you must examine what it is you are leading and the things you are trying to achieve.

Your aim should always be to put together a winning team who all get along with one another, who are all willing to work for each other, and who are all strongly motivated by your inspired leadership. Now might be a good time for you to revisit Chapter 8 *Developing the core values of your practice*, the values you are going to instil into everyone that works for you.

When you analyse your business there are several fundamental values that everyone working in your practice should embrace:

- employees
- quality
- patients
- continuous improvement
- communication.

Employee involvement is critical: success is a team effort.

Quality, that thing we all talk about but struggle to define: some people think of quality as being the standard of something as measured against other things of a similar kind, while others think of it as the degree of excellence of something. In your practice, who sets the 'quality' standard, is it the practice or is it your customers?

Patients are (and must be) the focus of every task carried out or performed in the practice. Everything must be done with patients in mind, providing better treatments and better services than other practices.

Continuous improvement is essential to the success of the practice: every employee must strive for excellence in everything: treatments, their value, patient care, competitiveness and profitability.

Communication, as I have said, is crucial.

Getting your employees to understand and appreciate the true significance of these core values is essential. Once you have achieved this, you can then start to develop a practice philosophy, one with real meaning and one that you can all espouse. It should incorporate all of the above plus anything else that you feel is important to you, your practice and your patients.

This was my practice philosophy:

The practice is dedicated to delivering service of the highest quality to its patients.

We place a great deal of emphasis on excellent communication, effective treatments and continuous professional development to enable us to completely satisfy our patients' needs.

Patients can expect to receive dental care of a high standard carried out in a calm, relaxed and safe environment.

It focuses on employees, quality, patient needs, continuous improvement, and the one thing that holds all of these together, communication.

You should try to come up with your own set of core values, and not simply pinch someone else's.

This practice philosophy is sometimes known as a mission statement or a statement of intent. Whatever you call it, you should display a copy in a prominent position in your reception area or waiting room for patients to see. Put a copy in each surgery and in the employee tearoom as a constant reminder to everyone. Make sure it's on your website.

As a practice owner and/or its manager, you have to be a leader. Leadership is never easy.

To me there are several key things that make someone a leader:

- they always focus on the positive
- they acknowledge the efforts of others
- they don't get bogged down by problems; they only see solutions
- they are very focused about what they want to achieve and are able to convey this to others

- they are innovative and are always looking for new (untried) ways of doing things.

Leadership comes from within.

Hold this thought: leaders have to pull from the front and push from the back.

(*See* 'Do you know where your practice is heading?' in Chapter 12 *Business planning.*)

Finding the (b)right people

Digressing from the military metaphor and Genghis Khan for a minute, in some ways building your team is similar to building a winning football team. Buying the right players, not just the best in the world, but ones who you think will blend in with the others at the club and whose style of play is suited to your vision, is the sign of a good football manager. One poor signing can disrupt the harmony of the team both on and off the field, and destroy seasons of careful planning. On the other hand, how many successful teams have fallen apart when their manager has left the club?

Leadership is easier if you have the right people around you and supporting you. Also, management is about getting things done through other people, so if you want things done right, get the right people.

Hold this thought: everyone you recruit must possess certain personal qualities and skills so they will be able to perform to the highest standards.

You want people around you who:

- are excellent communicators
- possess motivation
- are team players
- show a definite interest in self-development
- demonstrate that they could handle stress
- are able to plan and organise
- are good at using information
- can analyse and interpret information
- use their judgement when weighing up information and deciding on an appropriate course of action
- can make decisions
- use initiative
- can cope with changing situations
- understand the organisational environment of the practice.

This list of qualities and skills could equally be used to recruit someone to a senior post in a multinational company. There is no reason why you shouldn't look for the same qualities and skills in your employees, is there?

If you (or any of your employees) want to get things done through other people, it's important that you all are able to communicate clearly the things that need to be done. The ability to communicate is one of the most important skills you and your team must possess, not just the ability to communicate well with those within the practice, but also with those without.

Before communicating anything to anyone, you must have all of the relevant information, be very clear about what it is you are communicating, and know the preferred outcome.

Hold this thought: if you only have half of the information you can only ever communicate half a message.

To be effective, communication should always be short and simple. Brevity is a virtue. Communication comes in all shapes and sizes: body language (non-verbal), which includes gestures, posture and facial expression; verbal, which is almost always reinforced or negated by body language; and written.

It is a sobering thought that if your body language, tone of voice and your words are not saying the same thing, body language and tone will be believed more than the words you say. Face-to-face verbal communication allows both parties to observe each other's body language. The eyes give away what the mouth tries to hide. It is not only the eyes that reveal your true thoughts.

Verbal communication can be problematic because most of what people hear is forgotten, which is why misunderstandings occur. People retain little or only part of a verbal message and filter out much of what they hear. You have to repeat verbal messages if they are to be remembered.

Hold this thought: having employees who know the subtleties and art of communication helps build trust with your patients.

Being an excellent clinician is wasted if you lack the ability to communicate properly with your team and/or your patients. Similarly, surrounding yourself with a team of poor communicators is a recipe for disaster. Is poor communication inhibiting the performance of your practice?

Your employees must be able to work with others in a positive, cooperative and helpful manner. They should set an example through their own efforts for the team, and motivate others through their enthusiasm.

Surround yourself with people who actively seek self-development opportunities, and who want to reach their full capability in their current job and grow to their full potential.

A dental practice is a stressful place: stressed patients (adults and children), stressed clinicians, a stressed practice manager, stressed nurses and stressed receptionists. Your employees must be able to deal with stressful situations effectively, allowing work to continue, while they tackle the underlying problem(s).

Many of the skills and qualities listed above are those you would expect a good manager to possess. Should all of your employees be thought of as managers?

> I involved my employees in the day-to-day and some of the more strategic management of my practice long before it was an obligation under CQC. Now that employees are expected to know much more about the business in which they work, it seems that a great opportunity has opened up for them to take a more active role in helping to shape the practice, the way it is managed, and for them to personally improve their managerial knowledge and skills. Enlightened employers should embrace this idea and welcome any employee contribution, as long as it is positive, of course.

Not every new recruit will possess all of these qualities and skills. You must therefore learn to spot potential, especially in younger people, and be prepared to put time and effort into nurturing them to draw out their full potential.

Once you have assembled your dream team, your employees must 'wow' your patients with their professionalism, their friendliness and their expertise.

In a single-handed practice, if your nurse leaves you obviously need to replace them. But in a larger practice you might want to ask yourself, 'Do I actually have a vacancy?' 'Does the role have to be full time or could it be part time?' 'Is it a permanent job or would a temporary employee do?' Do you already have someone working for you who might like the job: a receptionist who wants to train as a nurse; a part-time employee who now wants to work full time? Don't rush into bringing in outsiders; redeploy your existing forces if you can so as to buy yourself time to find the right replacement.

Once you have decided that you do need to recruit (and this does not just apply to finding a replacement nurse) then you will have to:

- work out what sort of person you are looking for (does such a person actually exist?)
- decide how you are going to find them
- advertise
- draw up a shortlist
- interview
- appoint.

The person you want could already have either the necessary qualifications and/or experience, or you could employ someone with neither but whom you can train. This is time consuming, but it can be very rewarding. Qualified or not, work out the personal attributes your new employee must posses.

Your wish list of your ideal candidate might produce a person that simply does not exist, or if they do, could be too expensive to employ. Your ideal might have to be a compromise between what you'd like and what you can afford.

Bear in mind every practice in town is looking in the same places for their new recruits. So how do you gain an advantage over them and hopefully uncover someone that no one else has found? You could of course rely on an advert under 'Dental Nurse wanted' in the local newspaper, or you could contact the job centre or try dental recruitment agencies. Remember that now you have to be so careful about so many aspects of recruitment. (I am sure we've all heard stories of male dentists who claim that they will only employ glamorous females in their practice!) Then you have to ask yourself, 'Do I really need to spend money on expensive adverts that are probably not going to be read by the kind of people I want to work for me?' Why waste money on expensive agency fees? Why not look somewhere different?

You probably have lots of patients, some of whom will be school-leavers, who might be interested in making a career as a dental nurse. Your patients all have friends, relatives and neighbours who might be looking for a job in a dental practice as a nurse or as a receptionist or even as a practice manager. Make a mental note of anyone you come across who you think might fit into your team, and contact them if and when you have a vacancy. Get in touch with the careers advice teacher at your local high school and ask them to put anyone who is planning a career as a dental nurse in touch with you. Make and maintain contact with the nearest dental school; dental nurses wanting to move from hospital into practice, or student hygienists about to qualify, can all be pointed in your direction. Basically, keep your eyes and ears open for any prospective employees.

> Among my patients were several dental nurses and receptionists from other practices. Some of them asked me to bear them in mind if a vacancy ever came up at my practice. Here was a ready-made source of recruits.

However, if you decide to advertise you must make sure that the advert presents a picture of a professional and interesting organisation. Always check that your advert does not contravene current employment legislation.

At the very least the advert should briefly state the following:

- the duties and responsibilities of the job
- the qualifications and experience needed
- the personal qualities you are looking for
- the location of the practice
- an indication of the salary
- how anyone who is interested in the job is to reply
- whether further information is available.

You might want to draw up an application form and put together an information pack containing a copy of your practice brochure (they might be looking for a dentist even if they don't apply for the job) and a job description, which you can send to applicants. Always ask for a curriculum vitae and references (preferably two) from anyone who applies, because if you are going to attract the right calibre of applicants you must present a professional image, and that means going about things in the right way. Any time-wasters will not take it any further once they see that you run a professional organisation. Employment law is such a tricky area that you must not unwittingly lay yourself open to an allegation of discrimination from a disgruntled applicant. At this stage of the recruitment process, make sure that the same letter bearing exactly the same wording is sent to every applicant.

> I was caught out once by false references, so I would urge you to check, preferably in writing, the references of anyone you are thinking about employing.

A job description is an extremely important and useful document that you should give to every employee, but it is especially important when you are recruiting.

A job description should contain the following basic information:

- the job title
- the location(s) of the job (if they are going to work for you at more than one practice)
- who they are responsible to
- who they are responsible for
- the purpose of the job
- the main duties.

You might receive applications from people who have never worked in dentistry; do not dismiss them out of hand. In any case, you cannot discriminate against them for this sole reason. You should not restrict yourself to people who have only ever worked in dentistry, because you need to explore the possibility of introducing some fresh thinking into the practice, perhaps from people who have had a wide experience of working in customer care-related jobs. Don't be insular.

> I know a practice where the receptionist is a former manager of cabin crew personnel for a leading airline. She knows about customer care; it's such a shame the practice owner doesn't listen to her ideas and suggestions.

Interview all suitable candidates. Again, make sure that the same letter bearing exactly the same wording is sent to everyone you invite for interview. To avoid problems under the Disability Discrimination Act (DDA) 1995 it is wise to include a paragraph in the letter asking the recipient if there are any adjustments you will need to make to the place in which they will be interviewed. (It is unlawful for you or any other employers to discriminate against someone with a disability for a reason related to their disability.) Use a comfortable room for the interview and never rush proceedings. Be aware of your body language, posture, gestures, and watch theirs. How do you spot if someone is lying?

It is tempting to 'play it by ear' in an interview and to ask the candidates questions as they pop into your head. This is a dangerous strategy. Why? Again, it is all to do with discrimination and the employment laws. How can you reliably judge, compare and contrast the performance, responses and suitability of each candidate if you don't ask them exactly the same questions and score them accordingly?

Conclude the interview by telling them when you will contact them with your decision, which should always be in writing. Again, to avoid allegations of discrimination, I would always write the same letter to everyone who wasn't successful.

> I have been told by a reliable source that there are people who apply for numerous jobs and then, when they are told that they haven't got the job, lodge a claim for discrimination and seek compensation against the hapless employer. A cautionary tale.

Hold this thought: wherever you recruit from, never short-circuit the selection process, and always apply strict selection criteria.

Before you employ anyone, check the latest CQC guidelines and requirements, the person's eligibility to work in the UK, and don't forget to do an ID check.

Once you have appointed your new recruit you are legally obliged to give them a written contract of employment within a specified period of starting work. All of your employees must by law have a written contract.

Finding the right people can be a nightmare. The problem is that when one of your employees resigns you are then often panicked into having to find a replacement straight away.

I made some horrendous mistakes recruitment-wise, especially in the early days. I recruited one person who produced forged references, which I didn't discover until much later; one who I took on as a receptionist who said she could work chairside, but then when asked to help out in the surgeries refused; people who brought their domestic and personal problems into work; and one person who while she was supposedly on sick leave was actually working somewhere else. There are probably other examples that I have chosen to forget about.

I gave up using adverts and job centres; the quality of the people they produced was generally very poor. That's when I began to scout for potential employees among my patients and from anywhere other than adverts and the job centre.

The best team I ever had was in the last 6 or so years before I retired.

My practice manager/receptionist was a friend of my wife but someone I had never met; we bumped into her in the supermarket one day. She was looking for a job and I needed a receptionist. I interviewed her, obtained references and offered her the job. By the time she left the practice she had done every job except the dentistry! She learnt how to be a nurse and so took on the responsibility for training new nurse recruits. She ran the practice induction programme. She was a superb people-person; the patients loved her.

The receptionist had been my patient since I had taken over the practice. She was looking for a job and I was looking for a second receptionist. She'd never worked in a dental practice before but she turned out to be very efficient and also very good with the patients.

My nurse was someone who worked in a local café where I used to go for lunch. On this particular day I'd just found out that my current nurse had been working somewhere else while supposedly on sick. I jokingly said to the woman in the café, 'You don't fancy a job as a dental nurse, do you?' She replied, 'Yes please! I've always wanted to be a dental nurse.' She came to work for me and passed her nurse exams at the first attempt after a year of study. She loved her new career. She too was very good with people.

All three were technically very good at their jobs, but more importantly they were all mature enough to know that excellent customer care was what really mattered.

When you are looking for a receptionist or a new dental nurse it is worth remembering that dentistry is a profession, so the only people you should be interested in are those people who demonstrate a professional approach to their work. Employing people who do not take their work seriously or who show little respect for you, your work, their colleagues or your patients is a recipe for disaster. When you meet a prospective employee for the first time ask yourself, 'Do they look the part?'

I had a lot of dealings with solicitors and barristers in my capacity as an expert witness. I was always struck by the smart appearance, the nice way they spoke and the professional way in which receptionists, clerical and secretarial staff all conducted themselves in law firms.

Another thing to bear in mind is that all of your staff must feel at ease talking to a wide range of people from a wide range of social backgrounds. They must have an interest in the world around them, be able to talk about a wide range of subjects (not contentious issues such as religion or politics) ranging from popular television to sports, the arts etc. However, you must not employ someone who doesn't know when to stop talking.

Recruiting clinicians

The decision to recruit other clinicians should always be a business decision. There are advantages to having a large clinical team; there are also disadvantages (a large, unmanageable team?). However, while taking on an associate may not necessarily extend the range of clinical services the practice offers, employing a hygienist (or a therapist) certainly will. Dentists generally fall into two camps where hygienists are concerned: they either love them or they hate them. I am a great fan of hygienists and would advise any practice that can afford to employ one to do so.

Apply the same strict selection criteria when looking for a dentist or a hygienist or a therapist as you would when appointing any other employee.

A dentist, hygienist or therapist, as well as adding to the overall clinical expertise of the practice, must also make a significant contribution to the running costs and profit. Ideally you want them to also expand or 'grow' the practice. A rule of thumb in other professions is that whatever fees the 'employee' generates are split three ways: one third to cover the cost of employing them; one third profit for the business; and one third as their salary.

Once upon a time all associates were on 50%, that is, they received 50% of their gross fees after laboratory fees had been deducted from the top. There were usually no productivity targets, which meant that if a practice owner took on a low fee earner, then while the associate might not have been too concerned about their level of earnings, the owner, with all of the overheads to pay, probably was. On the other hand, if the practice took on a high earner everyone was happy. There are several ways to get round this problem of employing low earners, not only associates, but hygienists and therapists as well.

- Start them off on a lower pay scale, but offer them a bonus package based on their turnover and/or their profitability.
- Share information with them about the actual costs of employing them, in the hope that they then realise how much they have to earn for you.

However, creating an atmosphere in which you encourage high turnover creates its own problems and can lead to:

- a fall in the standard of overall customer care within the whole practice
- a fall in the standard of patient care within the surgery(ies)
- the possibility that clinical work is being done unnecessarily
- pressure on the practice's cash flow as more materials are being consumed and possibly more lab work is being carried out.

Then, how are you going to work out an individual clinician's profitability? If you can work it out, do they have to wait until the end of your accounting year before they are told the good or bad news? Will they trust your figures?

Your accountant should be able to help you work out if you can afford an associate, a hygienist or therapist.

Telling all of your employees actually how much it costs to run the practice and, if you feel the need, how much it costs to run each individual surgery, is one way of getting them to appreciate why earning money is important. If you aren't comfortable with sharing all of this 'sensitive' information with them, alternatively you could try this approach:

- work out, say, the cost of the telephones, postage, stationery, heating, lighting, water, waste collection, dental materials, and anything else you can think of, for a year
- present the figures to your employees in a meeting, but do not tell them what each figure relates to
- ask them to guess or work out which figure is which.

Not many, if any at all, will appreciate the magnitude of your running costs. Hopefully this will be a sobering lesson for them. You could ask them to compare these figures with their own cost of living figures; the problem here is that many young people still live with their parents and so might not have any idea about the true cost of running a house or a flat.

The topic of money is potentially divisive because your employees might not always appreciate working in a shabby practice for low pay, while all you talk about is your flash lifestyle. To them, the two won't add up.

Your practice needs to have a competitive edge, and so when you are thinking of recruiting an associate look for one who can bring additional or enhanced clinical skills with them.

I employed hygienists and, in the latter years, a therapist. The only time I didn't have a hygienist was when there were none around. I always felt that I was giving my patients a much better service and a much higher standard of clinical care if they were able to see a hygienist.

Over the years I had several associates. The principal/associate relationship is a strange one because as the owner of the business the principal quite rightly has the right to dictate how things should or should not be done, especially when they see something being done incorrectly. Some associates resent this and, as one particular recently qualified associate kept telling me, because they were self-employed and a qualified dentist, no one was going tell her what to do! We soon parted company. I had one associate who came from a hospital background. They were very good clinically, except that they took too long to do things, and they had absolutely no idea about the cost of materials or lab work.

If I were to go back into dentistry I would want any dentist who joined the practice to have a financial stake in the business. I think people's attitudes change when it is their money that is at risk.

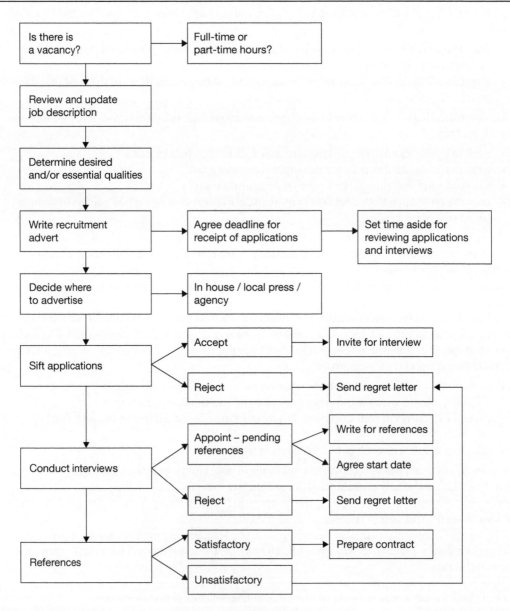

Figure 10.1 The employee journey: getting them on board

I remember a friend telling me that he'd gone for an interview for an associateship. This friend has a master's degree in restorative dentistry, but at that time he was simply looking for a job in a general practice as a general dentist, while he decided what he was going to do. Anyhow, the dentists interviewing him never asked about his postgrad degree, and when my friend mentioned it the other dentist responded by saying that all they did in the practice was 'ordinary dentistry', so it made no difference to them. My friend declined their offer of a job. Some practice owners fail to spot opportunities.

Managing the induction process

The induction process applies to everyone who comes to work for you, and that includes dentists.

Getting a new employee settled into their new surroundings and into their new job is something that should not be left to chance. It is in your best interest to help them integrate as quickly as possible and become as efficient and effective as soon as they can. Fail to do this and they can end up making erratic progress, but in the meantime costing you money, wasting materials, time and, at worst, possibly losing you patients.

Obviously the depth and breadth of any induction programme has to be tailored to the recruit's existing knowledge and experience, but it is vital that you educate them in the ethos, language and standards of the practice. This can quickly be done if you have a practice manual to give them on their first day at work, or even before they start work. Such a manual should contain information about the things they need to know. It can contain whatever you think is essential information, but at the least it should tell them about:

- the organisational structure of the practice
- the practice's mission statement/value statement/philosophy
- the practice charter
- health and safety issues
- data protection policies
- child protection policies
- your employment policies
- job descriptions for all roles
- policy on holidays
- sickness, absenteeism and lateness policies
- rules about employee behaviour and dress-code
- disciplinary policies
- grievance procedures
- how an individual's performance will be assessed.

I appointed a nurse from a practice not too far from mine: she seemed right for the job, so she came to spend a half day with us in preparation for starting work the following week. We talked about her work, how the practice was run etc. and I gave her a copy of the practice manual to take home and read. She looked at me in horror when she saw the manual; it was obvious that she'd never seen one before or had had to read about and understand a dental practice. She went home and phoned me to say that she'd changed her mind about taking the job. I was initially annoyed, but later realised I'd had a lucky escape; I wanted a dedicated worker, someone who was really interested in the job. Her current employer was welcome to her, I thought.

How to put together your practice manual is discussed in Section V *Policies and procedures*. You should break the induction process down into small, easy stages, for example:

- cover the bare essentials in the first couple of days
- the next 3 to 4 weeks should involve learning by a mixture of approaches, explanation, watching and practice. Be careful not to overload them with too much information

- during the next 2 months or so they should become totally familiar with your working practices.

The induction programme itself should include some fundamental components, for example:

- find someone who is willing to act as his or her mentor. In a small practice this might have to be you
- introduce the new employee to everyone in the practice
- emphasise the importance of the practice's policies and procedures
- allow them to give you feedback; you should be prepared to alter the induction process if things aren't going to plan
- always set out the standards you are looking for from the beginning.

Experienced recruits might feel that they already know how to do the job, but it is important that everyone goes through the induction process because you need to find out exactly what they do and don't know.

I wrote the practice policies and procedures so that I could then write a practice manual. (I didn't have a practice manager at the time otherwise I would have got them to do it.)

I wanted to set out everything that an employee should know about the practice. More importantly, I was tired of having to explain how I wanted things done to my existing employees and to new recruits.

Excellent managers are basically lazy people; they get everyone else to do all the work. They also find ways of avoiding having to repeatedly do some things.

Hold this thought: why not insist that new clinicians spend some time working in reception?

Working with associates

Wouldn't it be wonderful if your associate turned out to be a clone of you, someone who shares your passion for dentistry, your dedication to customer care, and *your* enthusiasm for *your* practice? However, despite your rigorous selection process, the person you take on turns out to be more Frankenstein's monster than doppelgänger, something created from everything that is bad about a bad dentist; a dentist who shows no urgency, a distinct apathy, a lack of care, and a general disregard for you, your patients and your practice.

What you need to understand is that no one who works for you is ever going to be as hardworking, dedicated and committed to the practice as you are. Some might come close, but only *you* will possess 100% dedication and commitment. If you happen to find a good associate hang on to them. If you find yourself saddled with someone who is doing harm to the practice, get rid of them.

Associates can be hard work for everyone: nurses who won't work with Dr X; receptionists who don't like the way Dr X speaks to them; patients who complain that Dr X always keeps them waiting and never seems to have time to explain things to them properly. I could go on, but I won't.

However, associates also have gripes about practice owners, I'm sure. Some of the most common ones probably are:

- poor working conditions
- lack of chairside support
- lack of support or guidance in clinical decision making
- expected to see too many patients in a day
- not enough work
- never enough materials
- equipment that is constantly breaking down and takes ages to repair
- no control over their own appointment book
- lack of administrative support
- lack of managerial support

- inconsistency with everything
- lack of respect from rest of the staff.

I'm sure every associate has their own tale to tell.

So how can you make your relationship with your associate or associates as harmonious as possible? The first thing to do when you first meet or interview them is be totally honest and upfront with them. Don't promise what you can't deliver and don't tell them that the practice has or does such and such when you know full well it doesn't.

Two examples of not being honest spring to mind. There was the practice owner who told me that he used rubber dam for everything (this was at a time when many dentists didn't even use rubber dam for endo!) and when I'd started working for them and asked the nurse for the rubber dam kit, guess what, there wasn't one. The owner had never used rubber dam in their life. The second example was a practice owner who told me he had a hygienist (a big plus in my book) and when I got there this hygienist seemed to have disappeared, if indeed they ever existed.

Try to establish some common ground: explore their thoughts about a wide range of dental issues, clinical and non-clinical. If you have any doubts about employing them, don't.

Lay your cards on the table about the culture of the practice, its philosophy, and the way patients are treated, in fact, about everything. You are looking for someone who isn't going to rock the boat, and definitely not someone who despite their obvious lack of experience thinks that they know more about dental practice than you do. That is never going to work.

Associates for their part must also be honest and upfront when applying for a job.

Cast your mind back to your days as an associate: make a list of all the things that were bad about the practice(s) you worked in; make a list of the things that were good. Can you arrange things in your practice that overcome the problems you encountered so as to make your associate's life easier?

My first weeks as a raw associate were a nightmare. I was thrown in at the deep end, with an appointment book that was too busy to cope with, working in a cobbled-together surgery with a straight-out-of-school 'nurse'. There was no induction process and neither of us knew where anything was or how anything worked, and still the patients kept on coming. Don't leave your associates to flounder; make them feel wanted.

Working with hygienists and therapists

At some point you might employ a hygienist or a therapist. You might have a direct access hygienist or therapist working in your practice. There must be a strong business case for going down either of these routes.

Looking at the situation where the hygienist is working solely for you, and where you've employed a therapist, how can you help to make this relationship work more effectively and efficiently, more productively and profitably?

I am told that most DCPs appreciate the value of teamwork. You should therefore include them in team meetings and involve them in any decisions about the development of the practice.

Having a full appointment book is obviously important to you as an employer; you like to know that the hygienist or therapist is making money for you. As a general point, their appointment book should be as well managed by the reception staff as you would expect yours to be. However, a full book is not everything. Think about your own appointment book: you probably like to have the odd free appointment available over the coming days or even the next week, so you can slot review or follow-up appointments in as the need arises. This is good patient care. Rather than the hygienist or therapist being solidly booked for weeks in advance, it is a good idea to have some time blocked off which is available for follow-up appointments – again, excellent patient care. Patients might lose impetus if they have to wait weeks for a 15-minute review appointment.

It is imperative that the hygienist or therapist receives a very detailed written prescription from the referring dentist, and you must see to it that they have adequate time in which to do what they are expected to do, and to do it well.

There are probably some dentists who employ a hygienist simply as a money-making 'cleaner', and who never give them the professional and personal respect they deserve. Treat the hygienist the same way as you would do any other professional colleague: listen to what they say, discuss cases with them, and make sure you are both 'singing from the same hymn sheet' when it comes to the treatment and future maintenance of patients.

> Whenever possible, I used to take a minute to go into my hygienist's surgery if they had a new patient or a patient who I sensed was anxious about seeing the hygienist. Together, the hygienist and I would quickly summarise the treatment plan in front of the patient, and I would make sure that what we discussed was done in a very equal and two-sided way. This helped reinforce the teamwork aspect of the hygienist's role in the practice and in the care of my patients.

Make sure that the hygienist or therapist works in a fully functioning surgery and that all of their equipment is as well maintained as is yours. Allow them time to sharpen their hand instruments, or if they'd prefer, allocate the task to another member of the team. Sharp instruments make for lighter work, making scaling easier for the hygienist, and much more comfortable for both patient and hygienist.

I keep returning to this, but communication really is important, between all three parties involved, the dentist, the patient and, don't forget, the hygienist and therapist.

Everyone likes their efforts to be acknowledged and rewarded. The occasional 'Thank you' from you won't go unnoticed, nor will the right level of financial reward for hard work and commitment.

Having a direct access hygienist working in your practice is slightly different to you employing a hygienist. They will most probably rent a surgery from you, and can obviously see patients without the patient having to see you or another dentist first. The rental cost of the surgery needs to be carefully worked out (you might want to talk to your accountant) and an agreement must be drawn up (you might want to talk to your solicitor) so that both parties know exactly where they stand legally, especially if things go wrong and the relationship breaks down.

The direct access hygienist can of course see patients from other practices, which raises the question of 'poaching'. Patients are free to go to whichever practice they choose, but it will do your reputation no good at all if you or your practice are seen to be encouraging other people's patients to switch to your practice. Very strict protocols about accepting patients and returning them to their practice (if they indeed have one), and for referring patients who haven't got a dentist, all need to be clearly set out.

The treatment coordinator

The treatment coordinator (TCO) is a fairly new addition to the practice team, but is someone who, if they are the right person and if they are used properly, can be a great addition.

What does a TCO actually do?

- They can be the first 'visit' for a new patient.
- They explain the treatment and the treatment plan recommended and drawn up by the dentist to the patient.
- They explain the different treatment options to the patient, and their cost and finance options.
- Their ultimate purpose is to explain the treatment to the patient and hopefully get a patient to agree to have treatment done, without the dentist having to take up his or her time doing this. If not handled right by the TCO, this can unfortunately sometimes come across as aggressive selling.
- They can deal with all the necessary paperwork.

If you are happy talking about fees with patients (many dentists aren't), and can do it so that on the whole they agree to have treatment, and if it does not take up too much of your time, perhaps you don't need to employ someone to do this for you. However, if you'd rather just get on with the dentistry, consider employing a TCO. Here are some of the things you need to think about before you employ a TCO.

- How are you going to successfully incorporate a TCO into your practice?
- Make sure that everyone in the practice knows what the TCO does.
- Give the TCO their own room in which to see patients. The room must be comfortable, with a large computer screen (or perhaps a tablet) on which the TCO can easily show patients diagrams and pictures.
- Employ the right person, someone who:
  - knows about dentistry
  - is a first-class communicator
  - is comfortable talking about money and fees to patients in an honest and open way
  - gets on with the rest of the team
  - is very well organised.

You will only know if employing a TCO has been a success by the number of patients who return to have their treatment completed. You will only know this if you know beforehand how many of them weren't returning and why. Maybe it wasn't *not* having a TCO that put them off, but something else?

Working with laboratories

Having an excellent laboratory as part of your team is a major bonus for any practice. You might think that all you have to do is prepare the teeth, take the impressions, and hey presto! a week later a beautiful piece of laboratory work appears for you to fit. You might think you're doing your bit, but what about the lab's point of view? Are there ways in which you could help them to help you?

Well-managed labs should have a booking-in system for all the work that comes into them. They will have carefully worked out how long any piece of work is going to take to turn around, but, more importantly, how long it takes a technician to do the required work to the standard you expect, which should be very high. Don't expect the lab to turn around your work in super-fast time, unless you are prepared to speak to them first and get their full agreement. Understanding their time management is obviously important, as is effective communication.

Most labs will understand when you have a case where work is needed urgently or needs to be back before the lab's normal turnaround. Prior planning and factoring in these timescales are an important part of treatment planning. Talk to the lab *before* you start your work, not during, and ask (never demand) if they can change their internal work schedules (without it adding to anyone's workload, which might affect the quality of their work). Booking in large cases, or cases where you know you need the work back quickly, helps alleviate many of the problems on both sides. You wouldn't expect the lab to cut back on the time they gave to a piece of your work because another practice wanted one of their crowns back in 3 days instead of 10, would you?

It is vital that you establish and maintain a good relationship with your laboratory. It helps if you also pay their bills on time.

It's always much better when a practice has a work logbook in which all work that is sent to the lab is signed out, and then signed back in when it comes back.

> I had a meticulous booking-out and signing-in system for my lab work. This system worked except when the nurse (I always made it their responsibility, not the receptionists) forgot to sign work back in. I'd make them ring the lab, but on the rare occasions this happened, 10 minutes later the work would miraculously turn up, having been found in a place it should not have been (the nurse also hadn't looked too hard). This was the only time I'd blame the person and not the process.

It may seem obvious, but always schedule your lab work to come back at least the day before the patient's appointment; 2 days is better still. This gives you time to check the work thoroughly (and query anything with the lab) before you have the patient sitting in the chair.

Your systems and processes for managing lab work should always work in conjunction with your laboratory's.

> I am told that those practices that tend to have continual problems with labs, regardless of who they use, are the ones that are poor at communication and who don't have even basic systems for managing their lab work in place. Many lab owners dread it when they are approached by a practice that says, 'We've tried lots of labs, but they all let us down.'

You would expect your customers (patients) to give you immediate feedback if something wasn't right in your practice. You want this information so you can improve. Laboratories, at least the good ones, operate along similar lines, so don't hold back from feeding back to them anything you think is going to help them improve.

> I preferred to use local labs, and I also occasionally liked to go and watch the technicians at work. Why not invite your technician to spend time in your surgery? An exchange of ideas and an appreciation of each other's working conditions is never a bad thing.

Nurses and extended training

A dental nurse now has the opportunity to do more than the dental nurse could ever do, say, 20 or even 10 years ago. They can now take post certificate qualifications in:

- oral health education (OHE), which includes fluoride application and impression taking
- dental radiography
- dental sedation nursing
- special care dental nursing
- orthodontics.

The first two of these are probably the most useful in general practice, but only if they are successfully incorporated into the day-to-day working of the practice. Several possibilities spring to mind.

- The nurse could give OHE talks in schools, and in doing so promote your practice.
- If you have a half day off each week, and your nurse doesn't, let the nurse set up a room where they can give OHE to families.
- If you have a separate x-ray room, the nurse can take radiographs while you use your time in the surgery to write up your notes, say.

> A good friend of mine set up what he referred to as a 'Preventive Dental Unit' (PDU) in an unused room in his practice. He kitted it out, and his nurse used the PDU to give kids and their parents oral hygiene advice, demonstrations, and dietary advice. My friend was one of the early adopters of preventive dentistry, and having a PDU proved a great adjunct to his philosophy.

Orthodontic therapists

If you do a lot of orthodontics it might be worthwhile employing an orthodontic therapist to assist you. Before you employ anyone you must, however, fully work through the benefits and whether or not it is going to be cost effective to do so. It might look nice having the name of an orthodontic therapist on a plaque outside your practice, but if they end up working as a nurse or as a stop gap on reception, you aren't really getting value for money.

Clinical dental technicians

If you are not keen on denture work you might consider employing or renting out a surgery to a clinical dental technician. As with hygienists and therapists, it needs to be an arrangement that works well for both parties and one that ultimately benefits the patients and your bank balance.

Managing peripatetic specialists

Using specialists in your practice, even if they only work for one session a week, requires careful management.

The first question to ask yourself is, 'What benefits, if any, is this person going to bring to my practice?' If you can't think of any, you probably don't need them. The next question is, 'How can I successfully integrate them into the workings of the practice?' This might seem an unnecessary question – surely they just work in a surgery like any other dentist? Let's think about this a bit more.

- Their surgery might need specialist equipment, instruments or materials. Will they be providing these themselves or will you be expected to, and who will be expected to pay for them?
- Will they be using their own nurse or will you let them use one of yours, and if so, have you got a spare nurse to give them?
- If they want to work outside of your normal working hours, is this feasible?
- Does this newcomer have a different booking system to yours? Perhaps they don't have fixed appointment lengths. Perhaps they will make their own appointments.
- Would your receptionist know what to do if one of the specialist's patients contacted the practice with a problem when the specialist wasn't working at the practice?
- Where are the specialist's patient records kept and who has access to them?
- How are their fees going to be collected and who is responsible?
- Perhaps the most important consideration is, does the specialist (and any staff they bring with them) share your dedication to customer care and service?

> I rented a surgery to a specialist who caused havoc at my practice. They were an excellent clinician but when it came to customer care they really couldn't have cared less. They ran over time all the time, keeping patients waiting without any explanation or an apology. My receptionist was forever having to make excuses. The worst bit was that the patients who had been referred from other practices thought that this was the way we dealt with all of our patients. Not good. Having an excellent clinician working as a specialist in your practice is not always the same as having someone who really cares about their patients.

Having anyone working at your practice, especially a fellow clinician, who is not on the same wavelength as you and your team when it comes to patient care, is very unsettling for everyone. Employees become anxious because they see things being done that they know shouldn't be done. Patients become anxious for the same reason. You risk losing good employees and patients.

Managing recruits from another planet

Your recruitment process should be such that whenever a new employee begins work there are no nasty surprises. However, it does not always work out like that. People who have worked at another practice might do things differently to how you want them done, or they might just not do things at all! Potential employees will sometimes tell you that they know how to do something when in reality they don't. Unfortunately, that's human nature. As part of their job interview it might be a good idea to ask a dental nurse to run through, say, a root treatment on molar, getting them to accurately describe the stages, the process, instruments and materials. A receptionist could be asked to say how they would handle, say, a patient who presented themselves at the practice demanding to see the dentist. Clinicians can be asked clinical questions *and* ones relating to customer care.

It is vital that you inculcate practice policies, procedures, and above all its culture, into new employees. Use a probationary period to identify any flaws in their character, any traits that you feel are going to inhibit the smooth running of the practice or introduce disharmony, or a lack of knowledge or understanding about what their role entails. Don't persevere with unsuitable new employees; life's too short and your practice is too important.

However, they might have simply been poorly trained or not trained at all by their previous practice, so don't be too hard on everyone who is at first not perfect. But do not put up with the employee who is constantly telling you how they did it at so-and-so's practice. Gently remind them that they work at your practice now and that you have tried-and-tested policies and procedures that they must now follow.

Recruiting people who had worked in other practices was always an illuminating exercise. 'Experienced' nurses whose knowledge of dental procedures and materials was rather limited; receptionists who thought good customer care was *not* snarling at the patients. Inexperienced associates who think that now they can get away with not doing many of the good practices they were taught at dental school, for example, not bothering to record BPEs, or not keeping even half-decent patient records.

If nothing else, taking on people from other practices gave me a great insight into what other practices must be like. However, now they work for you, they do it your way or not at all.

Employee records

You need to compile a personnel file for everyone who works for you. This should include:

- a copy of their original job application
- copies of references
- personal information, full name, date of birth and contact details
- immigration records and entitlement to work in the UK
- evidence of any professional qualifications they hold
- a copy of their current General Dental Council (GDC) registration certificate
- proof of current professional indemnity insurance
- their Disclosure and Barring Service (DBS) check
- their job description and details of any amendments
- salary
- pension details
- pay as you earn (PAYE) records
- objectives
- their performance reviews
- courses, training and personal development records, with copies of any certificates
- holiday entitlements
- sickness record
- disciplinary records
- a note of any practice property they have been given
- a record of whether they have been issued with any computer logons or passwords.

It is advisable to show the employees these records whenever an entry is made. Arguments can be avoided if your personnel files are kept up to date and are available for the employee to read.

Remember that under the DPA employees have the legal right to see any information you hold about them.

You currently have to retain PAYE records for a statutory period of 6 years. Data protection legislation and employment laws set out periods for the retention of data. Make sure that you always comply with current legislation.

Hold this thought: maintaining excellent records makes for an easier life.

Team building

Your team is one of the cornerstones of your practice, so building an excellent team is one of the keys to success.

Your employees will be more effective and efficient if they can be made to work as a team. Building a team, as opposed to just a collection of individuals, will:

- make the most of individual expertise and knowledge
- increase motivation and build confidence as individuals learn and feel more involved
- encourage collective problem solving
- help improve communication and reduce rivalry and point scoring
- encourage support for collective initiatives such as a patient care programme
- foster a climate of trust among employees, where mistakes are not punished but are seen as learning opportunities.

You should not have a practice that is 'us and them'. Arrange some 'out-of-work' activities (during working hours. People often resent being told they have to do work-related activities during their leisure time). Most of all, make your employees feel valued, which is one of the things a good leader should be doing.

> Team building might seem a bit passé, but it is very important. I was at a meeting with a councillor who had been drafted into our city's Health and Wellbeing Board, which is made up of people from a variety of backgrounds. The councillor told me that one of the first things they had to do was attend a team building day, at which one of the things they had to do was learn how to give and accept what might appear to be criticism from each other. The objective was to foster mutual respect.

There are several things that get in the way of building a good team.

- In larger practices barriers can develop between nurses who become territorial and protective of their 'little patch'. To stop this from happening, periodically swap the nurses around. You can sell the idea to them as it being part of their development, learning new work patterns etc.
- Individuals can lack respect for or understanding of how difficult another person's job can be. Make your nurse (and the clinicians, perhaps?) spend a day working on reception, or have the receptionist spend a day observing in the surgery.
- Dominant individuals deliberately try to exclude others from being part of the team; this is part of their little power games. You can either try to change negative behaviour or manage the individual concerned out of the practice.
- People coming from other practices can sometimes come with an 'I know best' attitude. Again, either work to change any negative behaviour or send them on their way.
- Sometimes people are simply not team players. Either you filter them out at the recruitment stage or lose them along the way. Either way, keep them out.

Objectives are a very good tool for managing employee behaviour.

In days gone by businesses operated with little or no input from their employees, other than what they were being paid to do. This changed as businesses slowly realised that they were not making the most of their employees' skills and experience. To get more from your employees you need to give them more freedom and responsibility to manage themselves, while still making them accountable for their

> One of the practices I worked in before I bought my practice had a great team, not by design, but by accident. There were six nurses, all about the same age and all from similar backgrounds. By chance they all got on really well at a personal level, regularly going out together at weekends and having lunch together in town. There was never any friction at work; they all helped each other and worked as a really good team.
>
> When I had my own practice I attempted to eradicate this 'us and them' attitude, so I periodically swapped my receptionist and nurse over, usually for 1 half day every couple of weeks. The receptionist trained the nurse and vice versa.
>
> Although this initially slowed things down a little, there were enormous benefits for me if one of them was off work for a short spell. It also genuinely helped each of them build respect for the work that the other one had to do. It is easy to find fault, but it is not always easy to do it better yourself.
>
> In larger practices there might be plenty of employees who can all cover for each other, but in smaller practices this will not usually be the case. Having employees who can job-swap is useful. Versatility is a great thing.

actions. Give them the authority to make decisions, but make sure that you clearly define the limits of their authority before doing so. Empower them. CQC means that employees have to be involved with the business in which they work: I think this is a good thing.

Hold this thought: your aim should always be to build or put together a cohesive team.

Personal development planning

If you are going to build a winning team it needs to be one that is constantly improving (in the same way as your practice must be constantly improving). That means that each employee must have a personal development plan.

Development is not the same as training or education: it is a broad, lifelong process of improving an individual's skills, knowledge and interests as a means of maximising their potential. You should therefore make the time to work with each employee and to help them to draw up their own personal development plan, which in outline should look at the following:

- where they are now
- their career goals
- the development needs that are going to help them get to where they want to be
- identifying their options for learning, which should address their learning style and the resources available both inside and outside the practice
- helping them monitor their progress and to periodically modify their plan.

Your most motivated employees are not always going to be the youngest ones; sometimes middle-aged women returning to work after raising a family can be driven by a sense of wanting to make up for lost opportunities. Harness enthusiasm and use it positively to reinvigorate other employees who have maybe hit a flat spot.

What sort of development should your employees be looking at? Once they are qualified they should be thinking about such things as customer care. Courses like this are usually taken as National Vocational Qualifications (NVQ) and to different levels of competence. These are usually completed in-house and involve compiling a portfolio based on real customer care experiences. They are neither too challenging nor time-consuming, but they can help employees gain or improve self-confidence,

> All of my employees were encouraged to take an NVQ in customer care. It made them think more about what looking after people was all about. Another, perhaps not so obvious, benefit was that because they did all of the work at work, patients were able to see that the practice was indeed focused on improvement. Win-win situation.

which is invaluable. Any development that helps your employees improve their interpersonal skills or their confidence with, say, computers, is certainly worthwhile.

There are other 'informal' development opportunities that you should consider. For example, take the case of a nurse who is excellent with adults, but who finds treating and generally dealing with children difficult. How could you improve their skills in this area? You could try to teach them yourself, or perhaps give them a book on children's dentistry to read, or, if you work near a dental hospital, you could arrange for them to spend some time in the children's department as an observer. If done properly, this is an excellent way of learning; it also tells your nurse that you value them and that you want them to be as skilled and competent as possible.

Unfortunately the opportunity never arose for me to send my employees to other practices etc., but it is something I would definitely do now.

Occasionally, I brought in a very experienced nurse, someone I knew from another practice, to give my nurse a bit of a refresher, coaching her in surgery management and chairside techniques.

You too should also consider spending time not only in other practices that are similar to yours, but also in ones that are not. You never know what you might learn. You could discover new ways of doing things.

Of course personal development also applies to you: update your professional knowledge as and when; refresh your interest and enthusiasm by exploring aspects of your work you'd not looked at for some time. Maintain a log of each and every bit of development you undertake, and show it to your employees as a way of motivating them.

Hold this thought: the days when you simply walked out of dental school with a piece of paper that proclaimed your capabilities, and that was that, are long gone.

The modern workplace is ultra-competitive and you need to continually upgrade your skills and knowledge, not just so you can move forward, but rather to stop yourself from falling behind. This applies to everyone else you work with and employ.

If an employee hasn't got any ambition or career goals, maybe you can inspire them and help them find that drive and ambition. That's what leaders do.

Evaluating training and development

Everyone likes to get away from the practice for a day; to start at 9.30 a.m. instead of 9 a.m.; to just sit and be talked at; and hopefully with a nice lunch thrown in. That's how most people see a training day or course. But you've probably had to pay to attend, and if you have taken your employees along as well, there are also their fees to pay. Then there's also the lost practice income. The point is, unless you clearly identify what the training and development needs are for you, your employees and your practice, you run the risk of wasting a great deal of time and money, and will in the end be no better off.

To avoid this, and before you sign up for *any* course, you must:

- define what you want any specific training or development to achieve
- set objectives so you know what is to be achieved
- make sure that everyone (if you are taking your employees along as well) knows what the objectives are
- devise a way of comparing results with objectives
- evaluate the delivery of the training or development.

At the end of most training days or courses delegates are usually given an evaluation sheet to give feedback. The usual questions they ask are:

- How do you rate the person delivering the training/course?

- Were the handouts and material appropriate?
- Were the physical surroundings suitable?
- How could the course be improved?

You should always provide feedback.

Employees should be asked to discuss any training or courses they have attended at the next practice/team meeting; this way you can assess its usefulness, and it is also an opportunity for the rest of the team to pick up the salient points.

> In my role as an expert witness I once gave a talk about dentistry to a group of clinical negligence solicitors. I prepared some hand-outs, which I'd spent a great deal of time editing and proofreading. Anyhow, the feedback after the talk was all positive, except for one comment from one of the solicitors that said that I should have numbered the pages! I can tell you that it takes a great of time and effort for any speaker to prepare for any talk or presentation, but the only way they can improve is by delegate feedback.

Managing your knowledge

Members of the dental profession have to do, and prove they have done, a large amount of continuing professional development (CPD). Managing this can be an onerous task if you don't keep on top of it. At the start of each year work out how much CPD you are going to have to do, what you want to do and then when you're going to be able to fit it all in. Not only is there a time element to all this, there is also a financial aspect as well, which you should have built into your annual practice budget.

If your practice is going to continually improve, which it must do if it is not going to lose ground against your competitors, you must be prepared to:

- deepen your knowledge and expertise in areas that interest you
- broaden your knowledge into areas that perhaps don't interest you as much. Don't ignore areas you don't like.

As far as managing the recording of your CPD goes, you can either rely on doing it yourself, or you could subscribe to an online service that not only does this for you, but which can also provide you with the learning material. How you do it is down to you, as long as you do it. Remember that your CPD must be verifiable.

> I was at a dental exhibition a couple of years ago, when I overheard a dentist ask someone manning a stand of one of the online CPD companies, if he signed up today to an online CPD service could he get 5 years' CPD credited by the end of the month? No was the answer. Obviously forward planning was not this dentist's forte.

Managing your clinical knowledge is something you will do almost automatically as part and parcel of your CPD. This is a very personal thing. However, as a practice owner, you should also keep your managerial knowledge up to date. What's the best way of doing this so that it doesn't end up taking too much of your time?

If you employ a practice manager, let them read and digest all the latest management information that comes into the practice, or which they come across during the normal course of events. Ask them to keep any very important updates, and then once a month, say, hold a meeting with them in which they brief you. Such a meeting need not last more than half an hour. This way you keep on top of things without having to expend too much time or too much energy.

Hold this thought: delegation is a key management skill, as is being able to identify and communicate only what is important.

Performance reviews (appraisal)

Reviewing or appraising the performance of your employees is something you should do at least once a year, but more often if necessary.

Why are appraisals important? The performance appraisal or review is not simply a meeting; it is an opportunity for you to discuss and evaluate the employee's performance as measured against their agreed objectives over a given period. It allows the employee to:

- have a very clear picture of what you expect from them
- discuss with you any concerns they have about their ability
- receive feedback and constructive criticism of their performance
- obtain your support and help develop their personal development plan
- be heard and respected.

For appraisals to be successful both you and the employee must:

- have a very clear understanding of the purpose and the process of the appraisal
- have a clear understanding of the terms of reference of the appraisal; if it is linked to a salary review, what criteria will be applied?
- prepare thoroughly
- decide how problems are going to be resolved.

You must allow the employee time to prepare by agreeing a date well in advance. You should emphasise to them beforehand that the meeting is not about apportioning blame if they have not achieved their objectives; it is about the two of you working together to remove any obstacles.

Having prepared, you now need to consider how you are going to conduct the appraisal. The meeting will be more productive if you:

- allow the employee to do most of the talking
- open by restating the purpose of the meeting
- reiterate that it is not about picking fault, but about helping them develop and improve
- encourage them to self-assess and to diagnose where the problems (if there were any) lie
- offer them support and help, but let them try to come up with the answers
- always try to be positive
- close the discussion by agreeing the areas where you both feel improvement can be made, and how any improvement can best be achieved.

Maintain good records of all appraisals, which should be filed in the appropriate employee file.

Performance reviews are good for many reasons, and you should aim to carry them out at least once a year. However, in a new practice you might want to keep a closer eye on how everyone is doing by holding them, say, every 3 or 4 months. This is fair enough except that your employees, who may all be new, might feel that they are being constantly watched at work. Strike a good balance between control and fear.

(*See* 'Objectives = appraisal' in Chapter 12 *Business planning.*)

Hold this thought: appraisal meetings help you engage with your employees.

Disciplinary procedures

Do you know how to handle a disciplinary problem involving one of your employees?

Are you up to date with the law on employee rights and unfair dismissal?

Management might be about getting things done through other people, but it is also about how you manage those people.

Hold this thought: good managers spot small problems before they become big problems.

You will need to keep your eyes and ears tuned to what goes on in the practice, but without getting sucked into gossip or tittle-tattle between the employees.

Having a formal written disciplinary procedure means that you will be able to deal with ill discipline in a structured and consistent manner. The procedure should therefore set out:

- definitions of the types of ill discipline it covers
- the presentation and documentation of warnings
- the rights of representation at disciplinary meetings
- time limits for investigation
- rights of appeal.

Before you start to write your disciplinary procedure try to obtain samples used in other companies or organisations. The Advisory, Conciliation and Arbitration Service (ACAS) should also be able to help you.

Most disciplinary procedures contain the following:

- an opening paragraph that explains why you have a written procedure, and why it is beneficial to both the employer and employees to have a set of rules for conduct in the practice
- a summary of the types of misconduct that would lead to disciplinary action – usually divided into two categories, minor and major:
  1. Minor could be such things as poor time keeping, not dressing appropriately or using a mobile phone at work.
  2. Major could include bullying, harassment, verbal or non-verbal threatening behaviour, fraud or theft, drug and/or alcohol abuse, inappropriate use of social media.
- the stages involved in the disciplinary procedure:
  1. oral (with written confirmation)
  2. first written warning
  3. final written warning
  4. dismissal.

The employee currently has the right to be accompanied at any disciplinary hearing by a work colleague or a union representative.

ACAS sets out current guidelines for disciplinary procedures and it is best to follow these.

Before you embark on any disciplinary procedure you must fully investigate the circumstances and gather as much evidence as you can. If you suspect that the matter might escalate it is advisable to seek professional guidance as soon as you can.

Don't lay yourself open to a charge of unfair dismissal by not following the legal protocols.

Grievance procedures

Do you know how to manage a work-related complaint from one of your employees?

You should set up a grievance procedure in a similar way to how you went about setting up a disciplinary procedure, so that employees have a way of bringing their grievances to you (or the practice manager). The law requires that an employer must inform their employees of the person to whom they can take their grievance and in what form it should be, e.g. verbal or written. ACAS will be able to provide you with all the up-to-date information regarding your obligations as an employer.

Try to obtain copies of grievance procedures from other organisations. ACAS is a good place to start.

Most grievance procedures contain:

- the types of grievances the process covers
- a summary of the stages that the process can go through:
  1. an initial informal meeting
  2. a formal meeting
  3. arbitration.

The initial informal meeting is an opportunity to resolve the problem, and you must give the employee the choice of discussing the matter with either you or the practice manager. One of you may be the person they are complaining about.

> Some employers do not know how to treat their employees properly. Others are not aware that it is not only *what* you say, but *how* you say it that matters. Inappropriate comments or suggestions do not make for a happy practice. But it is not all one-way traffic. One of my nurses came out with an inappropriate comment about me in front of a female patient. After the patient left I tackled the nurse about what she had said. The nurse left my employment soon after.

Conflict situations

When you are confronted with conflict at work do you shut your eyes and hope it will go away or do you encourage all parties to talk to try to resolve the situation?

Conflict between employees or between you and one or more employee is potentially destructive. Sources of conflict can arise between individuals because:

- they have a (strong) difference of opinion
- there is a clash of personalities
- there are problematic working conditions
- of unrealistic work expectations
- one person indulges in discriminatory behaviour
- there is poor communication
- there is non-compliance with the practice's values or accepted behaviour.

Try to head off potential conflict situations by learning to recognise when they might occur. Do this by listening to and observing behaviour. If you see a likely conflict don't turn a blind eye. If a real conflict does surface then:

- stay calm and take time to respond, but if tempers are running high give those involved time to calm down before moving on
- listen to *all* points of view
- avoid fight or flight
- stay assertive – which does not mean being aggressive, it means:
  1. acknowledging the opinions of those involved
  2. encouraging the identification of the cause(s) of the conflict and helping find the solution(s)
  3. finding a constructive way forward.

Conflict at work is never nice or easy to deal with. As the owner of the practice you have the final say in who works for you. If there is one employee in particular who is constantly upsetting others then take firm action (within the limits of current employment law) to remove them, but not until you have carried out an exhaustive investigation of the background.

> I always found having a more mature person as a receptionist worked well in heading off any conflicts between younger members of staff. The receptionist acted as a mother figure and was usually perceptive enough and experienced enough (having raised a family) to spot the first signs of trouble.
>
> I came across bullying behaviour in the first practice I worked in. Initially everyone got on, until the senior nurse left and was replaced by someone from another practice. This nurse then began to verbally bully a Youth Opportunities girl we had working with us. As if that was not enough, another of the nurses, one who had been nice to work with up until then, suddenly changed, and she too turned into a bully. The newest nurse did not stay long.

It is not always easy to spot bullies or potential bullies, but once bullying raises its ugly head it must be stamped out.

(*See* 'It's all in the mind' in Chapter 11 *The practice manager.*)

Employee absenteeism

How much time and money do you lose through employee absenteeism?

Do some employees resent having to regularly cover for a persistent absentee?

Do you overstaff to cover for absenteeism?

Are there any patterns of absenteeism?

The aim of managing employee absenteeism is to try to actively reduce it. By doing this you will:

- minimise disruption of the smooth running of the practice
- improve or maintain productivity
- reduce employee discontentment
- reduce the stress placed on you and the other employees
- reduce the risk of patient dissatisfaction.

When formulating your employee absentee policy you must first be aware of the legal framework. You cannot treat absenteeism due to genuine ill health as a disciplinary matter, nor can you insist that the employee takes the time off as holiday leave.

Before you can tackle unacceptable levels of absenteeism you have to define what those levels are. This will be expressed as 'more than X days in a given period'.

Keep records of absences. Employees are less likely to take time off if they know that you are recording and monitoring it.

Set out how and when you want absentees to notify the practice. If the practice opens at 8.30 a.m. you should expect to be notified no later than 9.30 a.m. on the first day of absence, with a reason for the absence and when they think they are likely to return to work. Employees should also be made aware that other notifications are required; for example, a fit note.

Some organisations hold 'return to work' interviews. These might be useful in protracted or persistent cases of absence as they allow you the opportunity to investigate whether the absence is likely to recur. However, any employee who has a long-term underlying health problem should always be treated sympathetically.

You can mitigate absenteeism by not recruiting poor attendees in the first place. Ask for references that tell you about their attendance record. Satisfy yourself that they are fit to work.

> I had a very reliable nurse until her partner returned from the army; she then started arriving late for work and would take days off when I was sure she was not 'sick'. Changes to an employee's home circumstances can change things at work. Keep your eyes and ears open about what is going on in your employees' lives.

Employee turnover

As much as you hope to have the same people working for you year after year, employee turnover is inevitable. If you are lucky and turnover is low, so much the better, but if you have a period when you just can't seem to retain anyone, you have to acknowledge that you have a problem. The recruitment process can be costly and time consuming. Another 'cost' is the effect this turnover can have on the rest of the team in terms of loss of morale, and on your patients, most of whom like to see the same faces every time they attend.

You must manage employee turnover in the same way as you would any other aspect of your practice. If you manage it properly it will lead to a more effective recruitment process and it will almost certainly help to reduce recruitment costs. It will also help to raise the morale of the remaining employees, which is very important.

As part of managing employee turnover, you should:

- establish the extent of the problem
- work out why people are leaving
- conduct exit interviews to find out why they leave
- look at the effect of employee turnover on the business
- look at ways of retaining employees.

People go to work for more than the money; don't think that you are necessarily going to retain them just by paying them more. People also need self-fulfilment. Employees leave for all sorts of reasons, but you need to establish whether or not there is an underlying problem with your practice, whether it be your working practices or a problem with one particular employee.

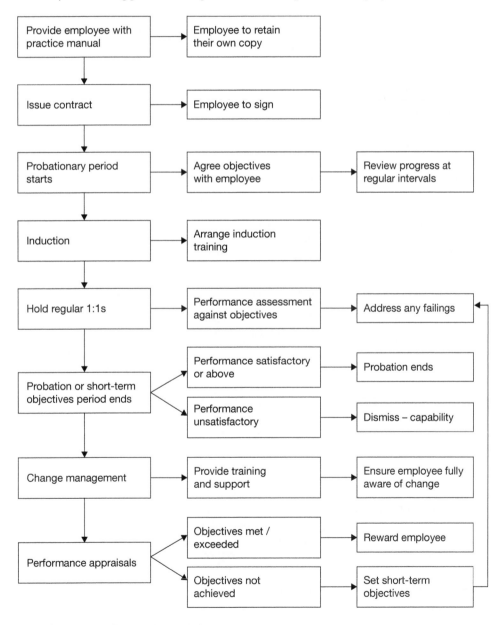

Figure 10.2 The employee journey: the travel plan

It could just have been my imagination, but periods of higher than usual employee turnover seemed to coincide with a lull in patient attendances. It was almost as if the patients could sense when there was disharmony within the practice.

If you want happy patients, get a happy team.

Employee departure

Whatever the reason for someone leaving your employment it is important that you follow a set procedure so that there are no loose ends. On their last working day either you or the practice manager should:

- ensure that the employee receives all pay due to them
- hand them their P45
- see that all practice property they may have been given is returned
- cancel any authorities they may have had, e.g. ordering from suppliers
- cancel any employer pension contributions
- cancel their healthcare/insurance benefits
- delete or suspend their computer access
- confirm their address so that you can forward their P60
- wish them well in their new job.

You might want to conduct an exit interview to find out why they are leaving. They of course might not want to give you the real reason, but if you have had a good working relationship with them they might tell you. It is important to know.

If the employee is someone you would be prepared to take back, say so; they may hate their new job.

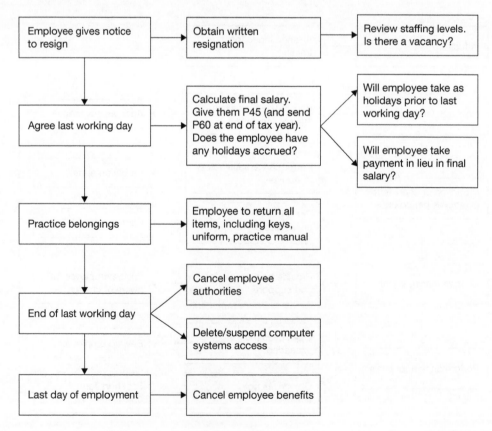

Figure 10.3 The employee journey: the end of the line

When an employee gives you their notice you should ask yourself whether there is a vacancy that must be filled. If you are not sure, have a go at working with the employees you have been left with for a short period to see how that works. Maybe you don't need to replace them after all.

The departure of a clinician

A clinician in this context is a dentist, a hygienist, a therapist, or a clinical dental technician.

When you lose a clinician, the big problem is what to do with their patients. There are a number of options depending on whether or not you are going to replace the clinician.

- The patients can 'return' to you.
- The replacement dentist or hygienist or therapist can take them over, either immediately, or after a short interlude if they aren't starting work for a while after the other clinician has left.

However, perhaps an even bigger problem might be finding a replacement clinician who is able to start work the day after the current clinician leaves (this is the ideal situation, but one that probably doesn't happen very often, I suspect). The smooth transfer of patients from the outgoing to the incoming clinician should not pose any problems if you can get the new clinician to start sooner rather than later.

You might have spent time persuading your patients to see the original clinician, singing their praises about how, for example, they really will be better cared for by the new hygienist. You might then have to back pedal a bit and persuade them that having their scale and polish carried out by you is not that bad after all.

If you manage to find a replacement, but they can't start for a month, say, this too should not pose too much of a problem. You might have to complete some treatments or just simply be on hand in case they have any problems in the intervening period.

You might have decided not to replace the clinician (maybe the experience of having them work in your practice was not that good after all) in which case you simply take over the care and treatment of the patients.

If it is a dentist who is leaving, do you ask them to complete all of their treatment plans before they leave, or do you have to sit down with them and work out a way of dividing their earnings up according to how much they manage to complete and how much they leave for someone else?

> At one of the practices I left as an associate I arranged to finish *all* of the ongoing treatment on *all* of my patients. This made for a nice clean break. There were no part-payments to negotiate.

Patients will always be curious about why someone is leaving, especially if it is a dentist or a hygienist or a therapist. If they have left on good terms, that is fine, but if they have left under a cloud make sure that nothing negative is said to anyone, which can be perceived as unprofessional.

Hold this thought: at the back of your mind you should always be asking yourself, 'How would I replace . . .?'

Getting the most from practice meetings

Whether you hold regular practice meetings or only have them when you or the practice manager feel that there is something important to be discussed with other employees, it is vital that the meetings are productive.

There is often the perception that meetings are a waste of time, that they are a breeding ground for resentment, and that they do not produce any meaningful decisions. This is more likely to happen if a meeting has no firm objectives, no agenda or there is a lack of leadership.

There are a number of tactics you can use to ensure that your practice meetings achieve results. You should:

- set very clear objectives
- decide who needs to be present
- pick a date and time that suits everyone
- set the agenda and circulate it to all attendees.

My practice meetings were always on a day of the week when every member of the team was at work and therefore could attend. We started first thing in the morning so no one had the excuse of running late with a patient if the meeting had been at the end of a session.

You may decide that you will chair all practice meetings, in which case your role is to:

- see that the meeting starts on time
- deal with routine items quickly
- introduce each agenda item and emphasise the objectives
- guide and control the discussions
- conclude by emphasising action points
- make sure that full, accurate notes are made, distributed and retained as permanent record.

Some employees might regard meetings as being an extended tea break or a way of airing their views or feelings about others. It is best, therefore, to adopt a business-like tone for the meetings from the outset. Don't allow verbose or opinionated members of the practice to dominate.

You may prefer to have a fixed agenda; one that is broad in content so that anything and everything you might want to discuss can be included. A fixed agenda will help to avoid anything being missed.

I would suggest the following agenda items:

- introductions and welcomes
- reports on any routine checks carried out since last meeting:
  1. clinical decision making
  2. protection of general health
  3. patient feedback
  4. personal development and training
- review of any patient complaints or serious untoward incidents since last meeting
- any difficulties encountered by practice members with working systems
- any suggestions for service improvement not already raised
- chairman's recap on any decisions taken about changing working systems
- time and date of next meeting.

These items are self-explanatory.

Any action points that come out of the meetings must be followed up by the person to whom they are allocated. If they are not followed up, nothing ever gets done.

'Routine' practice meetings should not overrun, but when more creative thinking is required a less formally structured meeting may be necessary. Meetings held away from the practice are often a better way of freeing up the creative thought processes.

I held practice meetings on a monthly basis and we always stuck to the same agenda.
  The meetings were an invaluable forum; we discussed and solved any problems the practice was having at that particular time.
  The most important thing was that action points were followed up.

It really is worthwhile giving up some of your clinical time to have team meetings. Once you get into the habit, and if they are well managed, these meetings are a great way of helping the team to gel, and of coming up with new ideas about how the practice can be made to work more productively and more cohesively.

Hold this thought: you don't have to do as much thinking if you get your team to do most of it for you.

Managing reception

Creating the right ambience in your reception area/waiting room is important. It is possibly the first contact people have with a practice and their experience will set the tone, and will be presumed by them to reflect the attitude of the whole practice.

A good receptionist must always be smartly dressed and must balance speed and efficiency with professional charm and sympathy. They should always be prepared to listen to talkative patients (people often talk more when they are nervous) but at the same time be able to continue with their work without seeming rude.

Your receptionist is a crucial element in the patient management process: *you* plan the treatment, decide what is to be done, how long is needed to carry out the treatment, and specify any intervals between appointments; the receptionist then takes over responsibility for patient management.

After the treatment has been completed the receptionist plays an important part in the review phase of the management cycle for any particular patient, particularly if problems had occurred. Perhaps laboratory work was not back in time because the receptionist had not allowed enough time between appointments (because the patient notes were not clear!). Or maybe you had not asked for enough time for an appointment (or the receptionist had to guess because the notes weren't specific enough!) and so your surgery ran late that day. This had a knock-on effect for the hygienist's appointments; many patients were kept waiting and some of them voiced their dissatisfaction to the receptionist.

To be an effective part of the patient management process your receptionist must be fully conversant with practice policies, for example:

- how you expect your patients to be addressed, either face to face or on the telephone
- how to handle patients requesting an emergency appointment
- when and how appointments are to be cancelled
- how to deal with patients who turn up late for their appointment
- what to do if you are running late
- what to do about failed appointments
- how to deal with patients who turn up without an appointment
- how to register new patients
- collecting payments from patients.

One other thing for which you should have an 'informal' policy is the circumstances under which you can be interrupted by a telephone call. This might be a simple 'Never!' or 'Only if such-and-such calls'. Your receptionist should know the rules and stick to them.

If you have decided that all patients are to be addressed by their title by the receptionist and nurse, and are only to be addressed by their first name by you and the hygienist, for example, then that is what should happen, every time. I have worked with young nurses who think it acceptable to address

I remember one day when a patient who lived on the other side of the Pennines failed to arrive for their appointment. It was not like them not to turn up. The waiting room was full when the patient turned up about 30 minutes late, full of apologies. An accident on the M62 had been the reason. I had a very good relationship with this patient and did not want to inconvenience them any more than they had unavoidably inconvenienced me this particular day. My receptionist had reviewed the remainder of the appointment book for that session, weighed up how we could still see the patient and still finish on time. With a bit of juggling, time management and cooperation from other patients, we saw the latecomer, carried out their treatment as planned, saw everyone else, and finished on time. Everyone was happy, including the patient whose 100-mile round trip had not been in vain.

older people by their first name even though they two hardly know each other. This may seem an old-fashioned attitude, but in a professional organisation respect is important.

Being able to deal with patients who are demanding to be seen even though they are late requires tact. The receptionist has to be able to quickly assess the situation (has the patient travelled far? Was the patient unavoidably held up in traffic? Are they normally good time keepers? These are questions the receptionist needs to ask themselves.) Set the rules, but give the receptionist permission to break the rules if necessary.

An excellent receptionist also needs to be:

- extremely well organised
- approachable and accommodating
- 100% focused on delivering excellent patient care
- confident, but not overconfident
- an excellent communicator
- prepared to make decisions based on a sound knowledge and understanding of your practice policies and procedures.

Once your receptionist has proved capable of managing reception and has earned your trust, give them total responsibility for its performance. Employees value being given responsibility and will rise to the challenge. They must, however, understand that they also have to take full responsibility for any mistakes.

The layout and organisation of your reception desk is not something that can be prescribed in a book like this; it is something that will evolve as your receptionist discovers what works best for them and for the smooth running of the practice. However, you should give the receptionist everything they need to carry out their role. Equipment must work or be repaired or replaced as soon as possible. Stocks of essential items such as notebooks, pens and pencils must be maintained. The receptionist must know how everything they are going to use every day works; for example, the telephone system and the computer.

Enrol your receptionist in a dental nurses' course at the local college; that way they can help out in the surgery if ever the need arises. They must also be willing to occasionally swop with the nurse to increase their understanding and appreciation of what goes on in there.

Your receptionist should be the epitome of efficiency, but they also need to be a people person.

Hold this thought: empathy, sympathy and understanding are key qualities in a receptionist.

A receptionist is also an intelligence gatherer. Patients will pass the time chatting with the receptionist, revealing information and valuable insights about themselves, their families, their likes and dislikes, all of which could prove useful when it comes to caring for and treating them, and for working out why they like coming to the practice. Some receptionists are very good at this. I came across one who used to read the 'hatched, matched and dispatched' columns in the local paper so that the practice could wish patients every happiness on their marriage, the arrival of a new baby, and to make sure that recall appointments were not sent to deceased patients.

The reception area can often end up as a meeting place for nurses when they have nothing else to do but stand around and chat. I didn't mind my staff doing this; however, I made it quite clear to them that when a patient approached or the phone rang, all talking stopped and the patient became the centre of everyone's attention. It's infuriating when you approach a desk, counter or whatever in any business and the staff, instead of welcoming you and asking how they can help, carry on talking about their night out or what they'll be doing at the weekend.

Managing the surgery

You spend most of your working life in your surgery so the last thing you want is for it to be disorganised and chaotic. The layout of the surgery is a personal matter; everyone works differently.

It goes without saying that your nurse must either be fully qualified or in training, and therefore will have a sound or basic knowledge and understanding of clinical dentistry. They must also be a good surgery manager so that it functions efficiently, which means that you are more likely to deliver treatments efficiently (and probably more effectively).

The nurse is responsible for the smooth, effective and efficient operation of the surgery; they must therefore be extremely well organised. Their management responsibilities include the following:

- patient care and safety in the surgery
- cross-infection control
- instruments
- storage and use of materials
- laboratory work
- stock control
- clinical waste
- patient records
- equipment.

Like an excellent receptionist, an excellent nurse must be:

- extremely well organised
- 100% focused on delivering excellent patient care
- approachable
- confident, but not overconfident
- an excellent communicator
- prepared to make decisions based on sound clinical knowledge and an understanding of your practice policies and procedures.

You and your nurse work very closely together and this relationship is one that needs to work in every sense of the word. Whenever you introduce new materials, techniques and treatments into the practice make sure that your nurse is made fully aware of them *before* you try them out on a patient. Rehearse new techniques and procedures, and iron out any problems beforehand (instruction sheets that come with materials or instruments are not always well written or correct). Nothing upsets a good working relationship more than having to correct your nurse because they have done something wrong, especially if you have to do it in front of a patient.

Your nurse must also know when to talk and when to keep quiet in the surgery. If you and your nurse must talk while you are treating a patient make sure that the conversation includes the patient, albeit as a passive listener.

Give your nurse total responsibility for the running of your surgery. If things don't run smoothly, at least you will see the gaps in their knowledge and training, which you can then close.

Your nurse must be willing to occasionally swop places with the receptionist to help improve the nurse's understanding and appreciation of what goes on in reception. The nurse must also be prepared to 'teach' the receptionist if the receptionist is asked to help out in the surgery.

> I liked to think of my practice as a small business made up of individual departments. I didn't have the time to manage each one on my own, so I gave the receptionist and nurse responsibility for managing their own 'department'. It worked.

Flexible working

This is not about the legal aspects of employees and their requests for flexible working; it is about you coming up with ways of making your practice 24-hour society friendly.

Being open from 9 to 5, Monday to Friday no longer suits the work patterns of the majority of people, so you need to think about how you can satisfy their demands for longer opening hours. To start with you have to have employees who are willing to change their existing work patterns. This is not always easy. You might have to recruit new employees to cover the extended hours, with all the training that that involves, and the extra cost.

Do you expect your employees (and that includes dentists, hygienists and therapists) to work all these extra hours? Businesses that operate as 24-hour, 7-day week concerns don't expect the same employees to work 24 hours a day, 7 days a week; they are run on a shift basis, and this is what you could think about doing. Begin by dividing up the working week into a number of workable shifts.

An example might help to explain how it could work in practice.

Four dentists, four nurses, four surgeries, all currently working a normal 9–5 Monday–Friday week, is a 35-hour working week (taking into account a 1-hour lunch break).

The practice, instead of opening Monday–Friday, decides to open its doors from 8 a.m. to 7 p.m., 7 days a week, but with no one working more than 5 days in any 7.

Dentists 1 and 2 start work at 8 a.m. in week 1, each has two nurses assisting in two surgeries. The dentists and the nurses do a straight-through 5-hour shift and finish at 2 p.m. Dentists 3 and 4 and the other two nurses repeat this, but work from 2 p.m. until 7 p.m. You will have spotted that each dentist (and nurse) is actually working 10 fewer hours per week, but the two-surgery arrangement makes them more productive, and being open earlier and later means they are likely to attract a lot more new patients looking for a dentist who can see them at a time that fits in more with their lifestyle.

In week 2, dentists 1 and 2 do the late shift and dentists 3 and 4 the early shift. In any 2-week period each dentist can book patients in from 8 a.m. to 7 p.m., and, with a bit of clever planning, from Monday to Sunday.

Obviously the nurses are not going to take a pay cut, so you will have to pay them the same for working 10 fewer hours per week, but as they are now working what many would consider unsocial hours, that's a decent trade-off. You will also have to compensate them for working weekends.

I would have at least three receptionists for this new shift arrangement: two working the shifts and at least one doing the core hours during the day. Continuity and communication are vital and must be maintained.

This new pattern of opening and working requires a great deal of planning, but it is possible.

Just before I joined the first practice I ever worked in the owner had the innovative idea of each dentist having two surgeries and two nurses. The nurses moved between the surgeries as they were needed, but whenever there was a patient being treated in a surgery there was always a nurse on hand to assist. The 'empty' surgery could be cleared, cleaned and set up for the next patient while the dentist attended their next patient in the other surgery. Productivity was greatly increased over and above the previous arrangement of one dentist, one nurse, one receptionist, and one surgery. However, excellent management of the appointment book became critical; such things as whether or not a patient required local analgesia had to be factored into the booking system.

Some years later when I had my own practice I modified this arrangement. I ran two surgeries, but instead of having two nurses and one receptionist, I trained all three employees to be nurses and receptionists. This system had several advantages.

o All employees functioned as nurses and/or receptionists. Holidays and absence through sickness were less of a problem because there was cover for all duties.

o The employee who assisted with a particular patient was then responsible for booking their next appointment. As the employee had heard all of the discussions with the patient they would know precisely what was needed.

o It promoted a great team spirit because it eradicated the divide between nurses and receptionist. If mistakes were made in the booking system it was up to the employees to resolve the matter themselves and to ensure that the same mistake did not happen again.

As I have already pointed out, with more stringent cross-infection controls these days I am not sure that this system of working would be possible. However, at the time it was innovative, and it certainly increased turnover and profit, improved my cash flow, and did a great deal to improve team spirit. Although I was working very hard it was probably one of my most enjoyable times in practice.

11

The practice manager

In an ideal world I think that every practice should have a practice manager so that the dentist can get on with the job of managing his or her patients and of earning money. Your practice manager might (have to) be you.

Practice managers come in all shapes and titles. The Association of Dental Administrators and Managers (ADAM) has listed 10 titles, which between them include the words 'Manager', 'Practice', 'Administrator', 'Business', 'General', 'Operations' and 'Development'. This range of titles demonstrates not only the potentially diverse nature of the post, but also how dentists and the post-holders themselves see the job. I will stick to using the title 'Practice Manager' throughout the book.

If you do employee a practice manager, don't let them just be a spare pair of hands in reception or the one who sends out the recalls. Your practice manager should be qualified and experienced enough to take on the role of 'manager' and all that that entails. If they have the experience but no formal qualifications, encourage them to take a practice management course. There are courses specifically for dental practice managers, but if you can't find one locally, or one that you think would be of real benefit to the employee or to the practice, consider letting them take a generic management course.

Many subjects can be studied as distance learning courses.

Even if your practice manager is a qualified manager you should still encourage them to continue their personal development by studying courses that perhaps are not directly related to management, but which in themselves can be of great value because they can help to improve their sense of self-worth and self-confidence. Don't rule anything out. You want a practice manager who is intellectually mature.

Your practice manager's knowledge should not be restricted or limited to dental management. Encourage them to look outside dentistry for their managerial know-how; for example, they could become a member of the Chartered Management Institute (CIM). They need to be prepared to expose themselves to as much management theory, practice and styles as possible.

> As part of my development and learning how to be a better manager I joined the CIM and went along to their meetings. I met managers from a wide range of businesses and picked up lots of useful management tips along the way which I could then take back and use in my practice. I even attended some of the CIM's courses and learnt about strategic planning, and basic management accounting.

If you are serious about your practice being managed professionally, why not look for a manager from outside dentistry? The business of dentistry is not that difficult or different that someone with the right managerial experience and knowledge should not be able to pick it up within a few months.

Whether your practice manager has been appointed from within the practice or has come from somewhere else, it is important that you give them the best chance of settling in and of finding out as much about the role as soon as possible.

The new practice manager must:

- learn as much about the job as they can beforehand
- gain as much from their induction as possible
- develop excellent working relationships with other employees; remember that if they have been promoted from within the practice, relationships may change
- aim to build a winning team

- familiarise themselves with suppliers and contractors and quickly build excellent working relationships with them
- be mature enough to honestly review their own progress
- learn from their mistakes and not dwell on them.

The responsibilities and duties of a practice manager will vary enormously from practice to practice, depending mainly on the size of the practice, and also on how much actual management responsibility they are given. There is, however, a general description that applies to all managers and that is that they have to decide what to do and then get it done through the effective use of the available resources. They should have the time to do all the things that you'd like to do to improve the practice, if only you didn't have to treat patients.

Hold this thought: don't pay a manager and then do the job yourself.

What are the functions of a practice manager? What things should you expect them to do and what should they be able to do?

ADAM very kindly provided me with a copy of what they regard as the competencies required from a dental practice manager.

- General management.
- Health and safety management.
- IT and technology management.
- Human resource management.
- Financial management.
- Physical resource management.
- Marketing services and sales management.
- Strategic planning.

All of these require specialist knowledge and expertise, and each one can be broken down and further expanded into a plethora of skills and knowledge.

Hold this thought: the practice manager's job is very demanding.

One characteristic differentiates the practice manager from other employees: they are privy to financial information and to ideas and plans before they are finalised and presented to others. Absolute confidentiality is therefore very important.

Remembering what the process of management is about, and no matter what they are doing, whether it be managing people, finance or facilities, the practice manager must always be able to:

- plan: decide on a particular course of action to achieve a desired result
- organise: gather together all of the resources that will be needed to achieve the result
- implement: get other people to work together smoothly and to the best of their ability as part of a team
- control: monitor, review or measure the progress of the work in relation to the plan and take steps to correct things if they are off course.

I think I read somewhere that the Japanese view of British management practice is that rather than following the Ready! Aim! Fire!' sequence, the British way is Ready! Fire! Aim! What the Ready! Fire! Aim! sequence really means is that people in general, and managers in particular, tend to take action immediately, reacting to something, before thinking it through thoroughly. You want a practice manager who is quick thinking, but not so quick that they take action based on incorrect assumptions or incomplete information.

Hold this thought: a cool head is better than a hot head.

As well as being able to be ready, aim and then fire, a good practice manager will need to possess the following qualities and attributes:

- a command of basic facts; they must gather facts before they act, not after
- relevant professional (managerial and dental) knowledge

- continuing sensitivity to events; correctly assess the changing lie of the land
- analytical, problem-solving and decision-making skills
- social skills and abilities; able to mix with everyone
- emotional resilience; handles pressure
- an ability to make things happen; proactive, that is, they must initiate positive actions that will benefit the whole practice
- creativity; come up with new ways of solving or doing things
- mental agility; able to juggle several tasks at once, i.e. multitasking
- balanced learning habits and skills
- self-knowledge.

Most practice managers climb up through the ranks, usually starting out as a nurse, then maybe 'moving up' to be a receptionist, until they finally reach the position of practice manager. There is nothing wrong with this career path, but it will only produce a competent practice manager if the holder of the post has assimilated managerial skills along the way. Knowing how the appointment book works or which firms you order your materials from is not enough. Next time you interview someone for the position of practice manager ask them what they did to market their previous place of work and how they went about formulating a strategic plan. Real managers will have the answers, whereas people who think that management is easy and therefore anyone can do it will struggle.

Many dental practices end up being 'managed' by the owner's spouse or partner, who may or may not have a dental or management background. I have no doubt that some of these managers are very good, but just because someone was once a nurse or happens to be married to the boss does not necessarily qualify them to manage a small business. It is far better to employ a professional manager, even if it is only on a part-time basis, who is more likely to give you impartial advice on how to run your practice.

> I have personal experience of three practices where the practice manager is the boss's wife. Not one of these women had any other management experience or qualifications, and looking back all three of them did nothing more than order materials and help out on reception.
>
> My wife was more than capable and well qualified to manage my practice (she was a bank manager with years of people management experience) but we agreed that she would leave the day-to-day management to my manager and me. I discussed broader management issues with my wife at home and would then discuss them again with the practice manager.
>
> At one stage I did employ an administrative assistant whose duties included managing the payment of invoices for materials and laboratory work, nothing too strenuous, but nevertheless important tasks.

Hold this thought: sometimes you need an outsider on the inside and an insider on the outside for balance, and to preserve your sanity.

What sort of management style will you be looking for from your practice manager? Their management style is the way in which they set about achieving results; it is how they exercise their authority, and it can be:

- autocratic or democratic
- tough or soft
- demanding or easy-going
- directive or laissez-faire
- distant or accessible
- destructive or supportive
- task orientated or people orientated
- rigid or flexible
- considerate or unfeeling
- friendly or cold
- keyed up or relaxed.

They must be able to strike the right balance between all of these styles, which should reflect the 'style' of your practice.

> What sort of manager was I? I was democratic, but autocratic when I needed to be. I was always demanding, but was aware that people didn't always understand or do things right first time. I was proactive, always taking the initiative. I was usually accessible and supportive, but only if the support was reciprocated. I like to think I was always people orientated, flexible, considerate, and I tried my best to be relaxed. Your management style should be a mixture of everything depending on the context.

The physical environment in which the practice manager operates is an important space. Everyone likes their office to be set out and arranged in a way that suits them. However, in a well-run practice the practice manager's office is the command centre, so some degree of organisation is important if the manager *and* the office is to function effectively and efficiently. (Don't think that you can stick your practice manager in a cupboard under the stairs with a desk, a chair and second-hand filing cupboard and expect them to manage properly – they need their own well-equipped office.)

Their office is where information from within and without the practice is received, processed, recorded, controlled and transmitted.

- Information is received – letters, telephone calls, faxes, emails, written notes, memos, verbal messages, computer data, verbal discussions.
- Information is processed – sorted and distributed for action.
- Information is recorded – classified, filed and recorded for future use.
- Information is transmitted – letters, telephone calls, faxes, emails, written notes, memos, verbal messages, computer data, verbal discussions.

Despite the fact that we live in a technological age, we do not yet live in a paper-free age. The filing cabinet remains one of the most prosaic and yet most essential pieces of furniture in any manager's office. Retrieval of the information stored in filing cabinets can, however, be a major problem if the cabinet is not well organised. Here are some tips on how to prevent papers disappearing into that black hole that is the office filing cabinet. The cabinet needs only three drawers, which should be labelled as follows:

- working drawer – this is for things that are ongoing, current year etc.
- A–Z drawer – this is for other things that are not necessarily being dealt with at the moment, but which need to be kept handy
- storage drawer – this is for things that are out of date or which are not used very often.

Use suspension files in the drawers so that papers can be stored easily and can be grouped together. Use the following system:

- broad, generic headings
- all headings should be nouns
- files should be arranged in alphabetical order starting at the front of the drawer
- the most recent papers should be at the front of a file
- papers should be cross-referenced
- never file papers that have paperclips fastened to them, that is how papers are 'lost' because they become attached to other papers
- if you reach the point where you think you need a bigger filing cabinet you are probably keeping too much paper, so go through each file regularly and dispose of unwanted papers.

The test of a good filing system is how quickly you can find something or, better still, how easily someone who does not normally use your filing cabinet can find something. How good is yours?

Files and folders kept on shelves should also be very clearly labelled.

You should only retain up-to-date and relevant paperwork, so periodically the manager should go through everything in the filing cabinet, remove unwanted or unnecessary papers and dispose of them appropriately.

> On the home front, my wife and I only keep what we have to, everything else goes straight into the bin or is shredded. Once a year we go through our filing cabinet and carry out a ruthless cull. Neither of us has ever later thought, 'I wish I'd kept that bit of paper.' The practice manager's office won't be big enough to store everything.

The practice manager, the great communicator

As I said at the outset, management has been defined as 'getting things done through other people'. It is therefore critical that the practice manager is able to communicate clearly the things that need to be achieved. The ability to communicate is one of the most important skills they must possess; not just the ability to communicate with those inside the practice, but also with people from outside as well. It is also one of the most important skills you and the rest of the team must possess.

Now we get to the heart of what being a great manager is all about.

But before communicating with anyone, the practice manager must:

- have all of the relevant information
- be clear about what it is they are communicating
- have an idea of the preferred outcome.

Hold this thought: to be effective, communication should always be short and simple.

> Maybe it's as I've grown older, or maybe it's because I'm not as patient as I used to be, but I like people to give me information as succinctly and as accurately as possible. I don't have the time to listen to or read waffle. Give me the facts, that's all I want.

However, most of what people hear is forgotten. The individual's capacity to remember information depends on how the information is presented. It may be no more than an urban myth, but it is often said that people remember 10% of what they read, 20% of what they hear, 30% of what they see, 50% of what they hear and see, 70% of what they say and write, and 90% of what they say as they talk their way through while doing something. Whether scientifically proven or not, this does give you some guidance about the best way to train your employees.

Hold this thought: the best results come if you get your employees to talk about what they are doing as they do something for the first time.

If you only ever tell your employees what to do or how something should be done, doesn't this explain why misunderstandings occur? People retain little or only part of a verbal message and filter out much of what they hear. Messages cascaded down, as well as those cascaded up, can easily be misunderstood. Misunderstanding grows while understanding declines.

> I was out having a pre-Christmas family meal. There were two menus available: the set price 2- or 3-course special, and the à la carte. Most of us opted for the special, but one of our party only wanted one course from the à la carte. Imagine our surprise when, as the waitress took our order, she told us that *everyone* on the table had to eat from the same menu, and that this is by order of the chef. Anyhow, after we made her go and ask the chef, we got the food we wanted. Thinking about it, this draconian order from the chef was ridiculous and simply did not make sense. What the waitress had been told was that diners could not, for example, have a starter from the special and a main course from the à la carte, no mix and match, which actually made sense. Either this had not been explained clearly enough to her or she had completely misinterpreted the instructions, or maybe it was a bit of both. Either way, the restaurant came close to losing several customers and a considerable amount in takings.

Quite often decisions are simply communicated or disseminated but not the information on which they are based. Employees will find it easier to accept and agree with a decision if they understand how the decision was reached.

Noticeboards are often misused; they should be the last place that an important piece of information is found. Talking of noticeboards: don't clutter up your reception area or waiting room with posters or notices stuck to the walls; people don't read them and it makes the place look untidy.

Cascading information downwards is obviously important, but feedback (communication) from everyone in the team about plans or proposals is also critical. However, feedback is naturally filtered (watered down) but the practice manager should nevertheless still try to gather it, otherwise it will stop being offered. If an idea from an employee is not appropriate, the practice manager must say so, but do it in such a way that it leaves the door open for the feedback to continue.

Hold this thought: if employees are continuously made to feel that their ideas are being ignored, eventually no more ideas will be offered.

There are a number of simple steps to improving communication within the practice.

- Simplify messages.
- Write them down if possible (verbal messages can often end up as a game of Chinese whispers).
- Repeat them.
- Allow questions.
- Explain decisions.
- Avoid notices.
- Only allow information to come from the correct sources.
- Set up regular communication/feedback (team) meetings.
- Be alert; be available to your employees and patients.

Very few dentists or practice managers are professional writers. For most, writing letters or communicating in writing is a chore. Scribbled handwritten referral letters, or a hurriedly signed letter riddled with errors, are sadly the norm in dental practice.

As with any piece of writing, if your practice's written communications are to be effective they need to be well planned. One method of ensuring that any written communication covers everything it is supposed to with nothing left out is to use Kipling's six serving men (*See* 'The practice manager as problem solver' in Chapter 11 *The practice manager*).

You do not have to use long sentences to say what you want to say. The English should always be clear, concise and correct.

When writing letters, if you address the recipient as 'Sir' or 'Madam' sign off with 'Yours faithfully'. If you address the recipient by name sign off with 'Yours sincerely'.

When you have finished writing you should ask yourself:

- Is the purpose of the communication clear?
- If I received this communication would its meaning be obvious to me?
- Have I left out any details?

As well as the communication within your practice having to be perfect, its communication with the outside should also be beyond criticism. I came across this in the first paragraph of a practice's website:

We are proud to be an (sic) Private Dental Practice long in (sic) the forefront of a movement to combine traditional high standards with a friendly approach which puts you first.

Now you might think, so what? It's the dentistry that matters! It does, but discerning potential customers are likely to steer clear of a practice that can't be bothered to make sure its website is error free.

What made things worse, when I clicked on the 'Our team' button on their page, it didn't work.

Get into the habit of double-checking every written communication you send and never sign one that contains any mistakes, no matter how trivial they may seem. Never let someone else sign your letters using 'pp'.

A signed letter should always be sent whenever you are confirming something or when you need a permanent record. Always keep copies.

Be aware that emails are generally not secure, and to comply with the DPA should not be used when sending sensitive or personal information. Encryption can protect data but it is complex to arrange.

Hold this thought: communication between everyone in the practice is essential, but remember that it is always a two-way process.

> Never underestimate the power of non-verbal communication. I was recently treated by a physiotherapist who had a couple of medical students with him. One of the students had their arms crossed during the whole session and even when they were asking me questions. To me this suggested that the student was being defensive or closed off. I would not want to see this if I was under the care of this person when they are a fully qualified doctor. People who never look you in the eye are often seen as being untrustworthy or disingenuous.

The practice manager as business manager

Leaving aside the question of whether or not your manager has the title of 'Business Manager', at some point you should expect them to draw up a business plan for the business. You should have a good idea of what a good business plan should contain from the time you put one together for your bank when you were looking to buy or set up a practice.

Although ultimately your practice business plan does rely on some input from the employees, a competent practice manager should be involved right at the outset helping you draw up the plan. They must therefore have a basic understanding of what a business plan contains and how to write one.

Basically, a business plan provides the means to:

- appraise the present situation of the practice
- appraise the future of the practice
- work out short-, medium-, and long-term objectives
- set out how those objectives are going to be achieved.

Remember that the business objectives must be supported by the personal objectives of the whole team.

The format of your business plan must:

- describe the ownership of the practice
- describe the background of the practice
- provide a profile of its patients
- contain a brief summary of the past performance of the practice
- give any key or major factors that will influence the future success of the practice
- define the objectives of the practice
- provide an analysis of the competition
- set out the practice's marketing strategy
- contain a financial plan
- set out a risk assessment.

It is not enough to know how to write a business plan; your practice manager should live and breathe every aspect of it every day.

(*See* 'Pulling everything together: your business plan' in Chapter 13 *Strategic planning*.)

The practice manager as marketing manager

Your marketing plan is part of your overall business plan. One of your practice manager's roles should be the successful marketing of your practice, which in its broadest sense means seeing to it that the services you offer are at the right price, are targeted at the right people, and that the practice is in the right place. Successful marketing is very closely linked with successful patient care.

Hold this thought: you can spend as much money as you want on marketing, but you should not have to spend anything if your patient care is perfect.

The practice manager can do a great deal of the groundwork beforehand to help write your marketing plan. For example, they can:

- assess employee skill levels that are going to give the practice a competitive advantage
- scan the dental press and look for new trends in products and services
- identify changing trends and tastes among your own patients
- make themselves familiar with trends in the local economy that may have an impact on the practice
- carry out a telephone survey of local practices to evaluate how well other receptionists answer the telephone, for example – do they sound friendly? Are they accepting new patients? Can you obtain practice brochures to compare with your own in terms of layout, general presentation and quality?
- develop questionnaires for patients asking them what they think of the practice, what it does well and what it could do better.

A questionnaire is an important tool in helping discover how you can improve your practice. With some planning and forethought it is possible to design your own questionnaire.

- Decide what it is you want to know.
- Decide what questions need to be asked.
- Arrange the sequence of questions.
- Determine how large the sample will need to be.
- Decide what you will do with the results.

> I am currently the chairman of the Patient Representative Group (PRG) at my GP practice. Every year the practice carries out a patient survey, which the PRG helps design. We try to remove any ambiguity and to ensure that we only ask what we want to know. Patients used to complain that the questionnaires are too long, so each year we play about with it, amalgamating some questions, removing others and generally shortening the whole thing.

You want to find out what your patients' expectations are in relation to the services and products you currently offer. It would be helpful to find out what expectations they have for the future.

Postal, telephone or personal interview research is expensive and time-consuming. Email might be easier, but you are then restricting your sample to those patients who have email. Are you going to hand the questionnaire out to every patient, or to every tenth one, say? Or is the receptionist only going to hand them out to those patients who they think will say nice things about the practice?

Placing the questions in the right order is important.

- Start with some simple questions that are easy to answer.
- Ask about current patterns/behaviour.
- Then go on to explore possible future behaviour.
- Follow a logical order to avoid confusion.
- Keep questions such as age etc. until the end.

How you ask the questions is important; for example, will they be open or closed? Responses to closed questions are easier to analyse, whereas those to open questions may provide more information, but will be harder and more time-consuming to unravel. Don't use technical words or jargon, which will only confuse the patients.

You will achieve a higher response rate if you keep your questionnaire short, make it easy to understand and very easy to complete.

Your practice manager should be able to design a questionnaire for you, carry out the market research and analyse the responses.

Market research is an invaluable management tool that you must use routinely to keep your practice on track.

Hold this thought: only by gathering marketing data and analysing it will you have the information on which critical business decisions depend.

If your practice manager takes an interest in marketing and shows any flair for the discipline, why not encourage them to become a member of the Chartered Institute of Marketing?

Membership of any professional, non-dental business-related organisations gives your practice access to information about what is going on in the wider business community. Membership of the Chartered Institute of Marketing will put your practice in touch with professional marketers who are at the forefront of current thinking about how businesses can promote themselves. Take advantage of other people's expertise.

I was a member of two management and one marketing institutes. I attended their meetings, mixed with non-dental business people and learnt a great deal about business in general.

Hold this thought: Genghis Khan used intelligence gathering as a strategic weapon; your practice should do the same.

(*See* 'Managing reception' in Chapter 10 *Managing employees* and 'Developing your marketing plan' in Chapter 15 *Marketing planning.*)

The practice manager as financial manager

A practice manager who is fully involved with the running of the practice, and who is not just a factotum, should have responsibility for managing the finances of the business. They are only able to do this effectively if they know how to draw up a budget and then, perhaps more importantly, how to control it.

Financial management is tackled in much more depth in Section IV *Planning*, but for now I want you to think about some of the ways in which a good practice manager should be earning their salary, not just by seeing to it that reception and the surgeries run smoothly, but by constantly maintaining and reviewing the financial information of the practice. Only by doing this are they are able to alert you to any impending financial difficulties. There are three financial indicators they should be monitoring: turnover; costs; bank balance (overdraft!). Let's examine each of these in turn.

- Problem: falling turnover.
- Causes:
  - decreasing amount of treatment being carried out per patient
  - losing patients (attrition)
  - failing to attract new patients.
- Solutions:
  - improve the thoroughness of each dental examination
  - take radiographs and check them
  - are recalls being sent out and what is the response rate?
  - contact every 'lost' patient and find out why they have not returned (very worthwhile market research)

- find out if there are any conflicts in the practice that patients might be picking up on.
  - review (or draw up) a marketing plan
  - observe employees at work; is complacency creeping in?
  - draw up a training plan to improve employee efficiency and to re-motivate them.
- Problem: increasing costs.
- Causes:
  - not sticking to budget
  - not having a budget in the first place.
- Solutions:
  - analyse every employee's contribution to the running of the practice; could some have their hours reduced, at least in the short term? Could others be dispensed with altogether?
  - find sources of cheaper materials
  - reduce stock levels
  - reduce the rate of consumption of materials by cutting down on wastage
  - cut energy costs
  - cut telephone costs
  - find a cheaper laboratory
  - draw up a budget.
- Problem: decreasing bank balance or rising overdraft.
- Causes:
  - falling turnover
  - rising costs
  - falling productivity
  - increasing inefficiency
  - practice expanding.
- Solutions:
  - see all of above
  - revise cash-flow forecasts
  - improve productivity
  - improve efficiency of the delivery of treatments
  - open longer hours (short term) to maximise the use of the equipment and the premises
  - call in unpaid patient accounts
  - contact creditors to gain more time to pay.

A practice manager needs to be a competent bookkeeper. Maintaining the practice 'books' is an essential element of helping to manage the financial aspects of the business. If this is an area where your practice manager is weak you could ask your accountant to recommend a training course, or they may even be prepared to train them themselves. There are online, distance learning courses you should look at.

The practice manager helping to increase profitability

Maximising the profit generated by your practice is an ethical as well as a business issue, but this should be one of your practice manager's key objectives. To maximise profit they must have a basic understanding of how profit is generated and how the things that contribute to profit interact. Linked to profit maximisation, on a day-to-day basis the practice manager should be discreetly monitoring the standard of customer care within the practice by:

- listening to how other employees talk to patients face to face and on the telephone – are they following agreed policies?
- observing how other employees interact with patients – what does their body language say?
- discovering whether employees are missing opportunities to 'sell' the practice to new patients?
- chatting to patients to obtain valuable feedback about how the practice is performing.

Has the practice lost, or is there a risk that it will lose, patients because the standard of customer care is slipping? Is a new recruit not towing the line and perhaps doing things their way? It is against this backdrop of constant monitoring of customer care that the practice manager then has to find ways of increasing profitability.

The practice manager should be constantly looking for ways to reduce running costs by cutting out or reducing a number of small costs as opposed to making one big cut to one cost, which is always more difficult to achieve. Anything, no matter how small its unit cost, should be trimmed back when profits need to be protected or increased.

> I'd had had my practice for about 3 years when I decided I must do something about my rising costs and a stubborn overdraft. I started in the surgery: I reduced the amount of stock, so eliminating 1 or 2 months' ordering; wastage was eliminated. I began to work smarter. In reception, patients were encouraged to settle their accounts at the start of treatment rather than at the end (and sometimes even later). Costs went down, money came in 1 or 2 months earlier, the overdraft fell and cash flow improved. Small changes to lots of things adds up to one big change.

Increasing the amount of treatment carried out does not necessarily increase profits, and the practice manager must be wary about encouraging the dentist or dentists to simply do more work (consistent with clinical needs). If you do go for growth, you must control your costs.

Hold this thought: profit needs turnover, but conversely turnover does not always mean profit.

> The principal of one of the first practices I worked in as an associate was constantly on about his associates doing more work, usually higher value crown and bridge work. That's all well and good, but doing more crown and bridge work simply added to his already precarious cash flow because the labs wanted their money months ahead of when the NHS would pay up. The practice turnover increased, but the cash flow worsened and, as the principal did not understand how money works, he simply encouraged us to do more and more work. While the practice's turnover increased, I doubt very much whether profit altered a great deal, if at all.

Are all of your surgeries being fully utilised? The capital tied up in each surgery must be used as much as possible so that it contributes towards the overall profitability of the practice. If you have a surgery that is only being used for part of the week could you rent it out to, say, a specialist who is looking to set up in the area, but who wants to test the water first before committing themselves to the expense of buying or renting premises on a full-time basis? Having a specialist within your practice could help to not only bring in welcome income, but it could also enhance your reputation with your patients. If done properly it can also be an excellent marketing opportunity.

> I have a farmer friend who knows the price of every bit of farm machinery. If he sees a combine harvester out on the road he can tell you exactly how much it is costing the farmer *not* having that harvester in a field somewhere earning its keep. Surgeries are no different.

Your practice manager should always be looking for ways to save you money, while at the same time looking for ways of increasing your income.

> At various times I had an orthodontist and a periodontist working at my practice. They both rented a surgery from me, but were both looking for their own premises in which to set up their specialist practices.
>
> I made sure that my employees knew what services the specialists offered and how these benefited patients. I also made sure my patients knew.

Hold this thought: put profit before patients and soon you'll have no patients.

The practice manager and time management

Your practice manager works very hard but is often complaining that there is never enough time to do all the things that need to be done. How can they get more done and avoid wasting time?

The effective and efficient use of your practice manager's time will ultimately have an impact on how much of the essential management of the practice actually gets done and how much is either left undone or forgotten about altogether. Excellent managers are usually excellent managers of time, and from your point of view it is in your best interest to have an excellent time manager helping you run your practice.

Here is a list of some of the problems that get in the way of excellent time management, together with some possible solutions:

- Problem: work piling up.
- Solutions: set priorities; set deadlines; don't underestimate the time tasks take (double your first guess).

Their work *will* pile up if they don't keep on top of things.

- Problem: trying to do too much at once.
- Solutions: set priorities; do one thing at a time; learn to say 'No!'.

Some people can juggle, but it is sometimes best to stick to doing one thing at a time.

- Problem: getting involved in too much detail.
- Solution: delegate more.

They should have a good overview, but do not always need to know the detail.

- Problem: postponing unpleasant tasks and procrastinating.
- Solutions: set a timetable and stick to it; do the unpleasant tasks first to get them over with.

We are all guilty of this, but it means that the unpleasant task gets in the way and stops you getting on with other things.

- Problem: not enough time to think.
- Solution: set aside blocks of time when there are to be no interruptions.

The manager must do, but they also need time to think, to plan.

- Problem: constant interruptions from people.
- Solutions: make appointments; set aside blocks of time when there are to be no interruptions.

The office is not a substitute for a staff room, it is a place of work.

- Problem: constant telephone interruptions.
- Solution: use an answering machine to field calls, and only call them back when it suits you. If your calls come via reception, tell reception which calls you will take and which ones are to be messaged later.

Control when to accept incoming calls.

- Problem: too much time spent in conversation.
- Solutions: keep to the point; learn how to end meetings without appearing rude.

Once you have the answer you want, stop.

- Problem: flooded with incoming paper.
- Solutions: sort papers quickly; use the waste paper bin; take the practice off mailing lists.

Control what comes into the practice and into the office.

- Problem: too many letters to write.
- Solutions: use the telephone more; devise and use pro forma.
- Problem: paperwork piling up.
- Solutions: do it now; use the first half hour of the day to deal with urgent correspondence; aim to clear 90% of papers each day.

- Problem: lost or mislaid papers.
- Solutions: don't leave papers on your desk; file them now; review your filing system; keep the office tidy.

Delegation is one way of managing your time, getting others to do things for you. The problem with this is that you have to keep a record of who you've asked to do what, and then you are relying on people doing things for you and on time, which doesn't always work.

Hold this thought: managing your time without setting priorities is like shooting randomly and calling whatever you hit the target (Peter Turla).

The practice manager as problem solver

The practice manager will be faced with problems every day and with everyday problems: some will be minor and easily resolved but others will require a great deal of energy and thought. If your practice manager develops a systematic and logical approach, the solving of *all* problems becomes much easier.

Rudyard Kipling wrote:

I KEEP six honest serving-men
(They taught me all I knew);
Their names are What and Why And When
And How and Where and Who.

This poem is sometimes called the journalist's questions; it covers every angle of anything you can think of and, what is more, when correctly applied it is infallible. Try it; it works!

- When you ask WHAT? you are looking for information about events, actions etc.
- When you ask WHY? you are looking for reasons, explanations etc.
- Ask WHEN? and you clearly want to know about times.
- Ask HOW? and you are looking for information about method(s) or processes.
- Ask WHERE? and you clearly want to know about places or locations.
- Ask WHO? and you want information about people.

Whenever you are faced with any work-related problem apply these questions and you will soon uncover the answers. Your practice manager should get into the habit of adopting this methodical approach to every aspect of their work, and these questions are a very good starting point.

> Once I discovered this lovely poem I used it all the time. It not only helps solve problems, it is also a great starting point whenever you tackle any task.

The practice manager putting things right

No matter how well your practice is managed things will sometimes go wrong. The practice manager must be able to identify the cause(s) and take the appropriate corrective action(s).

There are several reasons (nearly always people-related) why things go wrong and many more ways of putting them right. The most common reasons why things go wrong, with some suggestions how to put them right, are:

- an inability to learn from mistakes: mistakes are an opportunity to learn and to ask 'What went wrong?' Never make the same mistake twice
- incompetence: analyse the strengths and weaknesses of every employee; improve selection criteria; analyse training needs and introduce further training if needed
- overconfidence: employees who are overconfident tend to have tunnel vision. They believe that they know all the answers but do not take the time to see the bigger picture, i.e. what is going on around them. It is difficult to eradicate this problem

- underconfidence or lack of confidence: check to see that this is not incompetence; underline achievements and provide encouragement
- laziness: this cannot be tolerated
- lack of foresight: not thinking ahead leads to errors; plan carefully and learn from mistakes
- carelessness: due to overconfidence, pressure of work or thinking that a task is easier than it really is. Check everything!

Your practice manager must be able to quickly analyse a situation where things have gone wrong, and apart from rapidly putting things right, they must then take appropriate action to make sure that the same thing does not happen again. This may mean reviewing the level of training (or lack of training) of individual employees or of the team as a whole.

Hold this thought: getting to the cause of why something has gone wrong should never be a witch-hunt, nor should it be an exercise in blame.

The practice manager as health and safety manager

No practice management book would be complete without making some reference to health and safety, but this one will not attempt to cover the complex legal issues or give prescriptive advice.

Every practice must comply with the latest health and safety legislation: failure to do so can result in closure, fines and, in extreme instances, imprisonment. It is a serious business. Health and safety compliance is a component of the CQC inspection. You and your practice manager must therefore carry out a risk assessment, that is, the likelihood of an accident occurring, and then take appropriate action to reduce any risk.

By carrying out a risk assessment you:

- ensure that the practice complies with the latest health and safety legislation and by default CQC
- prevent accidents by identifying hazards
- show your employees and your patients that their safety is important.

The practice manager can carry out a preliminary inspection of the practice and identify any risks. These should include:

- fire risks
- manual handling risks
- chemical hazards
- risks from electrical appliances
- working areas
- noise problems from adjoining buildings
- chairs and desks
- computer screens.

Hold this thought: carrying out a health and safety assessment is all about controlling some of the risks in your business.

Information about current health and safety legislation should be obtained from the Health and Safety Executive.

Full-time vs part-time practice manager?

How much of the management of your practice do you want a practice manager to undertake? If you employ someone full time give him or her total responsibility for all of the management of the practice. If you employ someone part time you need to decide which bits you will give them and which bits you will do yourself. However, you could either share some of the work with them (if you like being a manager as well as a dentist) or you could employ an administrative assistant, who could pick up the less strategic management tasks, to work alongside the practice manager.

In a single-handed practice you could probably employ a part-time manager, but you would have to be prepared to take on at least some of the managerial tasks yourself.

Hold this thought: you cannot expect a part-time manager to manage a full-time practice full time.

Once a practice has more than one dentist I think you need to give serious consideration to employing a full-time practice manager, someone to oversee the smooth running of the practice. Full time or part time, they need to earn their salary, so I would set them well-defined objectives and link these to their pay or to any bonuses you might offer.

If you've appointed your practice manager from within the practice try not to let them forget their 'roots' and that they were once a nurse or a receptionist. It is easy for some people to forget that they once worked 8 hours a day at full stretch in the surgery or that they went home with a headache from talking all day on reception.

Hold this thought: a manger should never forget how hard other employees' jobs are, and that respect works both ways.

I'd like to end this chapter with a few words from an experienced practice manager, someone who has been there, done it, and has a wardrobe full of the tee shirts.

> The biggest challenge is not the patients, it is not even the dentists, it is the staff. No matter how big your practice might be, when you take someone on, you take on their family, friends, enemies, their good days and their bad days, in short, everything to do with that person. You have to be a sister/brother, a mother/father, an agony aunt/uncle, a counsellor, and a mediator.

> You have to be a diplomat, be a good listener and be prepared to own up when you don't have the answer. Managing good staff is the easy part; managing bad staff requires a good employment lawyer.

For much of my time as a practice owner I was the practice manager, mainly because once I realised how very important good management was to the smooth running of the business, I actually enjoyed the role. When I did employ a manager we tended to work in tandem, which for us worked well.

The type of person I would now look for, were I still in practice, would be:

o someone from a non-dental background, but who has a broad range of management experience
o intellectually mature
o extremely well organised, effective and efficient
o an excellent communicator, both verbally and on paper
o a team player.

I would not necessarily employ someone who had been a dental nurse and/or a dental receptionist unless they fitted the above criteria.

What would this practice manager do? The answer is: everything! So that I could get on with the job of looking after my patients.

It's all in the mind

Genghis Khan must have had his soft side, mustn't he?

It's all very well you and your team constantly striving for perfection (the perfect team; the perfect practice; the perfect everything) but it can and often does take its toll mentally. You might think you can cope running on full throttle all the time (some people think this is the only way to live), which is fair enough. However, as a responsible employer you should learn how to spot the signs and symptoms of stress, especially of stress overload, in your employees.

Hold the thought: the mental and psychological wellbeing of your employees matters.

Modern life is so full of pressures (real and imagined), big and small problems, hassles and niggles that you might have reached the point where you simply accept stress as a fact of life. Stress is now so commonplace that its signs and symptoms often go unnoticed, unrecognised, and sadly untreated.

Stress is a normal biological mechanism designed to protect you from harm. This is what is known as *fight or flight*. In a working environment, however, when you become stressed it is not always appropriate to fight (lashing out physically or verbally against the boss or a co-worker is not always a good idea), nor is flight (you need the job because you need the money). This inability to do something can lead to stress overload, and this is harmful. So what are the warning signs of stress overload?

The signs can be grouped under four headings:

- cognitive
- physical
- emotional
- behavioural.

Employees showing cognitive signs of stress often:

- have problems remembering things
- can't concentrate
- become very negative
- appear anxious.

Physically, employees can start to complain of:

- aches and pains
- frequent colds
- sickness
- dizziness
- in extreme cases, a rapid pulse or chest pains.

The physical expression of stress may not be so obvious to you, but telltale emotional or behavioural signs are not as easy to hide. It is changes in employee behaviour that you should be on the lookout for.

The employee who becomes moody or withdrawn, irritable or short-tempered, who bursts into tears at the slightest thing, these are all warning signs that they are not coping. They might suddenly appear to lose interest in their job and start to neglect their responsibilities.

It is never just one thing that makes someone suffer from stress overload. You've heard the saying 'the straw that broke the camel's back', well that is what happens with people. One day they are seemingly coping; the next, something else happens, which maybe on its own they could handle, and it all becomes too much for them.

Caring for your employees' psychological wellbeing is all part and parcel of your role. Being perceptive and aware of their moods, behaviour patterns and general demeanour right from the time you first employ them will help you pick up on small, subtle changes, which in turn should enable you to provide help and support. In extreme cases referral to a professional may be the best option for everyone.

Stress does not only occur at work, and the origins of stress overload may sometimes be at home. While I am not suggesting that you become a relationship counsellor or a psychotherapist, some understanding of the inner workings of the human mind is going to prove useful.

It is worth saying something here about bullying in the workplace. The purpose of bullying is to hide inadequacies, and therefore anyone who indulges in bullying behaviour is admitting that they are inadequate. This, however, does not help the person being bullied. Bullying destroys teams because it causes demotivation and disenchantment. If the bully is the boss they may achieve their goal(s) in the short term, but will never achieve any long-term success. The bully will try to isolate, subjugate and then eliminate the target. Their behaviour will be a series of small, often trivial incidents, which on their own won't attract disciplinary action, but when viewed and judged as whole often amount to a concerted campaign.

As the business owner you should never knowingly indulge in bullying behaviour, and you should always be on the lookout for signs of bullying within your team. If bullying does rear its ugly head you should take immediate action to eradicate it. Be aware that bullies are often well practised at deception and manipulation.

Bullies and bullying are a sad fact of life, and can occur at any stage in a person's life. Bullying is not restricted to any one social or educational class, so bullies may be respected people who hold positions of responsibility within their organisation or in society as a whole.

> One dentist I briefly worked for indulged in bullying behaviour, although I doubt he would see it as that. He used to call his nurse derogatory names in front of patients. The point here is that to him it was probably no more than a joke, but subconsciously it must have made him feel like the big man, being able to treat her in this way. His patients, rather than seeing him as the cultured, sophisticated professional (which he always liked to see himself as) will have seen him as a small-minded, uneducated bully.

If you suspect that bullying is taking place in your practice don't jump in straightaway; slowly gather evidence so that when you do decide to act you have a strong case for disciplinary action. The person or persons being bullied will need your support during the process, but if they are worth keeping they are worth supporting.

Managing management consultants, coaches and business advisers

You might at some point want (need) to bring in outside help, either for a short-term one-off project, or on a long-term ongoing basis. Consider these people to be your employees; after all, you're paying them.

There's an old joke that a management consultant is someone who will borrow your watch to tell you the time, and then keeps your watch. Seriously, management consulting focuses on the analysis of existing organisational problems, before coming up with a plan or plans for improvement. The aim is to help an organisation improve its performance.

Coaching is more about the individual, helping them achieve personal or professional goals. Coaches often ask questions that are designed to help the individual find the answers themselves.

Business advisers are more often than not people who have run their own business and who are now working to help (young) businesses get off the ground.

You are not likely to need all of the above at the same time, but you might call upon them at different stages in your practising career.

Add into this list 'mentor', someone, usually a friend, who guides a less experienced person by building trust and encouraging positive behaviour, and you have just about every stage of your business career covered. In your younger days you might turn to a dental friend or colleague for guidance about your career. You might, for example, want to explore various career pathways, as an associate, moving from an associate to practice owner, whether or not to specialise etc. Older, more experienced colleagues can be great mentors when you are just starting out.

> I have mentored several young dentists. It is a very informal arrangement, meeting over a meal and drinks, and them asking lots of questions. While it's always a compliment to have others ask for your views and opinions, I was aware that any 'advice' I gave had to come with a caveat. What worked for me might not necessarily work for someone else.

You might consider using a coach after you've been in business for a few years, as a way of refocusing your personal and professional goals, and when perhaps you've become a little stale. A coach should not want to get involved with the business process side of things; that is the management consultant's territory.

Management consultants, or at least the very good ones, usually come into their own when a business is having problems, so there seems little point engaging them if there aren't any problems. However, no matter how well your practice is managed there might be times when outside help may be needed, for example:

- if you recognise that the practice has a problem but has insufficient resources to resolve it
- the symptoms of a problem obscure its cause, which can only be revealed by a completely unbiased, objective examination carried out impartially by an outsider
- a conflict of ideas or views exists in the practice and independent assessment is required before agreement can be reached on how to proceed
- there is a lack of expertise within the practice.

Sometimes a fresh approach can stimulate the practice into thinking in a different way about its business, its operation or which way forward. Innovative ideas or a devil's advocate approach introduced from outside may have a stimulating effect.

> Some practices I have come across jump from one consultant or coach (some people don't know the difference) to another, desperately seeking the magic bullet to solve their business problems. The offices of these practices often contain numerous consultant reports, which have usually not been read more than once, if at all, and whose recommendations have certainly not been implemented. The problem these practice owners have is not only with their business, but with their unwillingness to listen to advice.

The term 'management consultant' is not a protected term, so literally anyone can describe themselves as one. Before you engage any management consultant carefully check their experience, qualifications and their track record of success. Ask for references, not only from satisfied clients, but perhaps also from unsatisfied clients. Make your own mind up as to whether the consultant is worth employing. Don't get swept along by the cult of personality or the flavour of the month.

Before you approach any management consultant you must have a very clear picture of what you hope to achieve. Choose one who is a member of a recognised professional body, membership of which is based on the consultant's professional knowledge and on their knowledge of the consultancy process. Contact professional organisations for a list of suitable consultants. Try to choose a consultant who has relevant knowledge of the dental industry, although in reality any intelligent consultant should be able to quickly learn how the business of dentistry functions. The question then is 'Do you want them to learn at your expense?'

Before you engage a management consultant I would recommend you find a copy of *Managing Consultants: how to choose and work with consultants* by Igor S Popovich. Read it and arm yourself with inside knowledge about:

- the games consultants play
- how to find the right consultant for the right job
- monitoring and controlling consultants.

This book will also show you how to get the most for your money by ensuring that the work they do for you is done on time and within budget.

Hold this thought: it is often said that a management consultant is someone who comes in to solve a problem and stays around long enough to become part of it.

Sadly, I have seen examples of consultants announcing to the world via social media that they are going to or have just been to such-and-such a practice. Would you really want everyone to know they'd been to your practice, and to perhaps incorrectly infer that your business was having problems? I wouldn't. Always build a very strong confidentiality clause into any agreement you have with any external adviser.

Occasionally you might want or need a practice manager but not someone permanent, or to bring in a manager for a one-off piece of work, e.g. compliance. This is when the interim manager comes into their own as they can provide a short-term or temporary solution when additional management skills and resources are needed.

Interim managers are useful for a number of reasons, but you should only ever pay them based on results (which means you have to set them very SMART objectives; *see* next chapter) and not on attendance. People often work as interim managers because they prefer to work in different businesses rather than in one. They often like the challenge of adjusting to new situations quickly or they prefer the flexibility. An interim manager should always bring professionalism and expertise to their job.

Hold this thought: if you are struggling, think about bringing in additional expertise.

Using clinical coaches

If you can bring in managerial expertise to show you how to improve the management of your business, why not think about doing the same to help you improve your own clinical expertise, someone with these skills who is prepared to give you hands-on, in-situ coaching?

> The principal of a practice I once worked in decided that perio was the way to go, but he had had no additional training, nor could he afford the time or the money to obtain the additional knowledge he knew he needed. He found a periodontist (I think they worked in a hospital) to come to the practice and show him how to examine for perio, how to diagnose, and how to draw up a perio treatment plan. This was in the days long before basic periodontal examination (BPE), when perio examinations were practically non-existent. This specialist spent several weeks with the principal. I don't know how much this clinical coach received in payment.

There are numerous areas in which you could improve your clinical expertise, and perhaps you don't need to learn more than the tricks of the trade, those little tips that can make you a slicker, more effective and better clinician.

> A young colleague and friend of mine has developed his expertise in the use of composites. I have seen some of his work, which by any standard is superb. He knows exactly how to handle the material and how to get the best results from its use. If I was in practice I'd be picking his brains to find out how he does it so that I could improve my composite restorations in my patients.

Why not investigate how you can improve your clinical skills and give your practice a clinical competitive advantage?

Hold this thought: if you aren't continuously improving you will soon fall behind.

Managing the boss

So far this book has been aimed at the practice owner and by proxy at the practice manager. The focus has been very much on how to build an excellent team from the top down, but what can or should the employee be doing to build that same level of trust and understanding with the practice owner? This subsection is meant to be read by employees; its purpose is to help you – the employee – build an excellent working relationship with the practice owner.

If you simply think of your job at the practice as 'a job' and you have no feelings of allegiance to the boss or to your colleagues, and no ambition to progress with a career in the dental profession, don't bother reading on. On the other hand, if you like working at the practice and you want to do well in your chosen career, what I have to say is hopefully going to be of some value to you.

Getting on with your boss on a professional and a personal level is extremely important if the workplace is to be somewhere you want to be.

There are a number of areas that can help you build this relationship:

- communicate effectively with the practice owner to prevent misunderstandings
- work out what is important to them
- support them in what they are trying to achieve. If you can't, maybe it's time to find another job. Loyalty is valued by employers and will eventually be rewarded
- clarify what they expect from you
- be confident in your work; this way you will be valued
- always present a professional image; dress smartly, smile and be positive
- don't harbour resentment; tackle conflicts in a mature way.

Your boss must be someone you get on with on a personal level. He or she must also be someone you respect professionally. Bearing in mind that you probably spend more time at work than you do at home, you need to help create a great working environment.

Dentistry stopped being a cottage industry a long time ago. It is a highly regulated profession, and practices have to have dedicated, hard-working people working for them and in them. Practice owners are under enormous pressure from all sides and will not only expect but should also demand the highest standards, both inside and outside the workplace, from everyone they employ. As an employee you owe it to yourself and your employer to aspire to the highest standards.

Hold this thought: as an employee working in a professional environment you must have the desire to learn and continually improve.

Section IV

Planning

12

Business planning

To extend the military metaphor of Genghis Khan at the head of his Mongol hordes, managing your practice is very much like leading an army. If you and your practice are going to survive, you and your employees must all be heading in the same direction, with the same objectives and with the same strategy. There will be times when you may be staring defeat in the face, when you have to reduce your fighting force and regroup. You may from time to time have to resort to guerrilla tactics to preserve the integrity of your army. You must know the type of terrain you are fighting on and what the enemy plans to do next.

This next section is your battle-plan, and as the Roman writer Vegetius said, 'If you want peace, prepare for war.'

I have come across practice owners who 'just want to do the dentistry' and who seem quite happy to leave the management and development of their practice/business to a third party. Practice owners, and the extent to which they are involved in the management and development of their business, fall broadly into three groups:

- those who are fully involved (always the best option)
- those who are never involved (a dangerous strategy)
- and those who might sometimes be involved.

Which group are you in?

Those who are involved must know how to manage. Those who are never involved risk everything if they rely on others, without the tools in place to retain control. Those who might sometimes be involved are the same as those who are fully involved in that they also need to know how. It's amazing how many practice owners think they can abdicate responsibility for their business to a practice manager and yet remain in absolute control.

Hold this thought: control is the central message of this book.

I liken managing a practice to leading an army. The analogy is not as strange as it might at first seem. Delegating management responsibility does not mean abdicating leadership. Defining your practice's purpose, setting its business objectives and formulating a strategic plan should all be *your* responsibility, albeit shared. If you have a practice manager you will of course involve them, and you will also have to involve your employees if you are all going to be heading in the same direction.

Hold this thought: leadership is a management skill you not only must learn, but which you must also be prepared to exercise.

From now on I talk about involving your employees as a way of helping you produce a better, workable mission statement, objectives (business and personal), business plan and a strategy. However, it is important that you still retain control of the whole process by, first, coming up with your own plans and, second, not conceding too much ground when others don't agree with you. You have to tread a fine line if you want your practice to be successful.

Hold this thought: involve your employees while at the same time remaining in control.

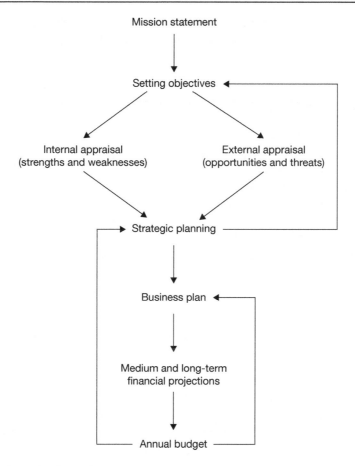

Figure 12.1 The business planning cycle

Do you know where your practice is heading?

'Would you tell me, please, which way I ought to walk from here?'
'That depends a good deal on where you want to get to,' said the Cat.
'I don't much care where . . .' said Alice.
'Then it doesn't matter which way you walk,' said the Cat.
'So long as I get somewhere,' Alice added, as an explanation.
'Oh, you're sure to do that,' said the Cat, 'if you only walk long enough.'

(The Cheshire Cat in Lewis Carroll's *Alice's Adventures in Wonderland*)

Not only do you and your employees have to be heading in the same direction, you all need to have a very clear idea of where you want to end up. You and the practice cannot possibly know how it is going to get there (wherever that is) unless you have clearly defined the destination.

Producing what is commonly referred to as a mission statement is the first step in this process of defining the destination. Whether you call it a 'mission statement', 'business philosophy', 'business values', 'practice purpose', 'statement of intent' or to use CQC's term, 'statement of purpose', is irrelevant.

Your 'mission statement' (I'll stick to calling it this) is important because it combines the inspiration of where the practice is going, how it is going to get there, with the realities of where it is now.

Some dentists seem to have a very clear vision of what they would like to achieve, i.e. where they are going, from very early on in their careers. Others seem to drift through their career, letting life take them to wherever it happens to take them. I am not saying that one approach is fundamentally better than the other in terms of happiness, but you are more likely to do the things you want to do and to be a more fulfilled person if you set out with a clear vision. Things may not always turn out the way you want them to, but I think it is still worth having a vision.

Why is having a mission statement important?

Your mission statement is important because it:

- will outline clearly the direction in which the practice is moving
- should provide inspiration for your employees
- will provide a definition of success
- will identify in what business the practice will be in the future
- is a living statement, which you and your employees can translate into objectives and goals for every aspect of the practice's operations.

A mission statement is a critical element in the strategic planning framework of your practice. Formulating your mission statement is often the first step when cultural changes are being introduced.

Hold this thought: a mission statement on its own does not create a sense of 'mission'; that can only come from you, the practice owner, and the inspirational leader.

Begin by deciding where you want the practice to be in, say, 1 year and in 5 years' time. (The objectives you set and the strategies you pursue are going to enable you to get there.)

In a single-handed or small practice you should try to involve all of the employees. In a larger practice you should initially limit it to those who have managerial responsibilities. You can then involve everyone when you have a fully thought through plan.

Embarking on the business planning process can pose a number of challenges for practices. You might find it useful to appoint an outsider to help with the process if, for example, there is:

- a conflict of ideas or views within the practice and an independent assessment is required before agreement can be reached on how to proceed
- a need to introduce fresh thinking or innovative ideas.

Once you open Pandora's box and start talking to people within the practice about mission statements (and everything that inevitably follows on) you might sense a degree of resistance (some people have an inborn fear of things they don't know about). As a first step, you should have found out as much as you can about everything that makes up the business planning process, so you are to some extent able to answer any questions. Some people may put forward different ideas or views: don't overreact when people disagree with you; again, arm yourself with the information you need to support your side of the discussion.

You might have got to this stage and have recognised that something needs to happen to the practice, but you don't yet exactly know what that something is. Don't struggle on; think seriously about bringing in outsiders, experienced professionals with the right background and qualifications, to help introduce fresh and innovative ideas into the discussion.

> Through my membership of the Chartered Institute of Marketing I came into contact with professional marketers. I engaged one of them to conduct an appraisal of my marketing plan. I was not averse to using outside help from time to time, even though I felt that I could do it myself.

Before you can decide where you want the practice to be at sometime in the future, you will have to assess where it is now. In determining this you will need to consult with your employees and also try to elicit the views of your patients.

Set aside time to talk to your employees, first as a group and then individually so that you can find out their views and opinions about the practice. Young or new employees may be very shy about telling you what they think. You will have to reassure them that you are genuinely interested in their views and that anything negative they say will not be held against them. You should make it clear that you want them to contribute towards helping to improve the practice, and that in the long term this will be for their benefit as much as for anyone else's.

> You and your employees inevitably have different perspectives of the world and of life in general, and about work and the practice in particular. You should not expect your employees to see things in exactly the same way as you see them. Someone once described dentists and practice owners as being concerned with numbers, while their employees are more interested in feelings. Bridging this gap between yourself and your employees is not impossible; it is all part and parcel of being an inspirational leader.

Try to find the areas that the employees agree on and the areas where there is disagreement. Try to get your employees to articulate their views clearly, and don't settle for 'I don't like it' or 'That won't work'. Ask them 'Why?' Have they any strong opinions about where the practice should be in the future? If their opinions differ widely from your initial thoughts, ask yourself, why? Are they right? At this stage you must have an open mind. Sometimes a thought or idea, no matter how strange it seems, opens the way for new ideas. Creative thinking is called for.

Receptionists are an invaluable source of information regarding what the patients think about the practice. Patients will say things to them that they would not say to you. (*See* 'Managing reception' in Chapter 10 *Managing employees.*)

> Sometimes it is the patients who can keep you informed about what your employees are getting up to out of earshot. I had a very disloyal and disrespectful receptionist at this time, and one day one of my oldest and, as it turned out, very loyal patients asked the nurse to leave the surgery; they went on to tell me what the receptionist had been saying about me and the practice. The receptionist probably thought that if I couldn't hear this I would never know. I confronted the receptionist, and after other incidents came to light, dispensed with their services. This person then had the cheek to give my name as a reference when they applied for another post. They must have thought I was stupid.

The most important part of your practice is your patients. It is stating the obvious to say that without them you do not have a business. You must find out what they think about the practice. Why do they come to you rather than go to anyone else? What do they like about the practice? Perhaps more importantly, what are the things they do not like? People naturally shy away from asking for feedback, either because people might think they are fishing for compliments or because they are afraid of hearing anything bad. You must not be afraid of asking patients for their opinions, good or bad.

Hold this thought: patient feedback is a crucial part of developing the practice.

Once you have collected the information from your employees and from the patients, you will then have to compare their views. Are they different? If so, why? Use the information to begin to build an overall picture of the practice. Resist the temptation to ignore any bad bits; eliminating the bad bits will help turn the practice into a super practice.

Discuss the findings with your employees and reach a consensus on a clear vision for the practice. It is crucial that you all share the values that you are evolving if the final mission statement is to have any real value and meaning. There may be obstacles to some of the things you are hoping to achieve, so you will have to explore people's resistance and try to overcome it. One way of overcoming resistance is by putting yourself in the other person's shoes, trying to see things from their point of view, understanding their motivation. One common obstacle which many people express concern about is that they feel that they lack the core competencies to enable them to handle their role within the 'new' practice. Different ways of doing things or doing different things altogether present challenges to everyone. You will have to reassure them that although change will be inevitable, it is something that you can all work through together.

Hold this thought: part of your role as a leader is to show and give support.

Your mission statement, and inevitably your mission, will fail if there is a lack of consensus. You cannot push ahead with your plan if you don't take everyone else with you. Sometimes you will have to pull from the front and sometimes you may have to push from behind.

You are now ready to draft a mission statement. Writing a good mission statement can be extremely difficult.

- It has to be specific without being too restricting.
- It needs to be flexible and adaptable but should not be changed every year.
- It should be inspirational but not unrealistic.
- It should be easy to understand but not simplistic.
- It should be based on patient need.

To help you write yours, bear in mind that most mission statements contain a reference to:

- aiming to be the best
- identifying the importance of people
- quality
- service
- communication.

You may like to remind yourself of my practice's philosophy, which in reality was our mission statement.

'The practice is dedicated to delivering service of the highest quality to its patients.

We place a great deal of emphasis on excellent communication, effective treatments and continuous professional development to enable us to completely satisfy our patients' needs.

Patients can expect to receive dental care of a high standard carried out in a calm, relaxed and safe environment.'

It focuses on employees, quality, patient needs, continuous improvement, and the one thing that holds all of these together, communication.

Above all, your mission statement must be believable. It should be worded in such a way that all of the employees can relate to it. However well it is written, your mission statement will fail if you do not convince everyone in the practice that you genuinely believe in it, and make them understand why you are pursuing that particular mission, and also what they are going to get out of it.

Hold this thought: experience has shown that the very best mission statements are the ones that have an emotional content – that is, they have captured the imagination of people.

When my practice started to become more patient-focused I needed to consolidate this major cultural change. Coming up with a mission statement was the first step. I didn't produce it on my own; it was something created by me, my practice manager, the hygienist, the receptionist, and the nurse. We all played our part.

It would be wonderful if all you had to do was write a mission statement and your practice then became a business with (or on) a mission. It takes much more than that. For it to work you and your employees have to wholeheartedly embrace its core values. Shared purpose, commitment and belief in what you are all trying to achieve is vitally important.

Taking time to produce a mission statement that is a model of clarity, succinctness and memorability is time well invested. If it is something that you and your employees genuinely believe in and are proud of, put it on your website, incorporate it into your practice brochure, your practice manual, and display it in the waiting area for everyone to see. It should act as a constant reminder to you and your employees.

Get it right and you have a good marketing tool; on the other hand, if what you produce is not worth the paper it is printed on, it will have completely the opposite effect.

Having decided on the general direction in which you want to set off, you now have to think very clearly about the places you want to visit. This 'map' is your objectives.

(*See* Chapter 10 *Managing employees.*)

Setting objectives: for the practice and its people

If your mission statement represents the general direction in which you want to guide the practice, your objectives are a more focused statement of your aims. You should think of an objective as being an end towards which the effort and resources (human and financial) of the practice are directed.

Objectives are important because without them your practice will lack the framework that defines what is expected from everyone and what is to be achieved. It can lead to your employees becoming confused and demoralised. People prefer to have clearly defined goals rather than some nebulous, ill-defined idea. For you, as the practice owner and leader, if you fail to manage by objectives, you risk:

- not knowing where the practice is going
- never knowing what the practice has achieved
- not knowing whether what you are doing fits into some long-term plan
- becoming confused and demoralised because you feel as if you have little or no control over your life.

Hold this thought: without objectives the practice will lack direction and purpose.

(It is very important at the outset to realise that an objective does not set out how something is to be done, it simply states *what* is to be done.)

Objectives must always be SMART if they are to be of any value.

- Specific (S)
- Measurable (M)
- Agreed (A)
- Realistic (R)
- Time-bound (T).

The acronym SMART is a good starting point when you are drawing up objectives. However, other properties or features should also be included to increase their relevance. They should be:

- well-defined
- positive
- achievable
- challenging
- written down.

Hold this thought: woolly words never achieved anything.

During the process of setting objectives, you must first set overall objectives for the practice – your business objectives. Your business objectives should follow on naturally from what has been said before about formulating your mission statement. Business objectives are normally related to financial management, i.e. income and profit, but you should also include other factors such as quality, customer care and employee development. Employee (personal) objectives are part of the next stage. Once you begin to think about the make-up of your objectives you realise that almost every aspect of the practice has to be included.

Test every objective you set against the parameters of SMART. Reassess your mission statement in light of the objectives. Do they complement each other or are there discrepancies?

An objective must always be in line with the core values of the practice as set out in your mission statement.

Hold this thought: once these have been set you can then begin to involve your employees in setting their own personal objectives.

Involve your employees

As the owner of the business, and therefore the one who presumably has the most to lose if it fails, you will set the business objectives. However, as mentioned previously, the cooperation and support of your employees is crucial if you are to have any chance of success. You should therefore 'share' the business objectives with them, while taking care not to allow them to exert too much influence over their final form.

Share your vision with your employees (individually and as a group) and encourage them to contribute ideas and suggestions about how the practice should (can) be developed. Certain people may have to be convinced about the value of having objectives and may have to be encouraged to meet those which they feel are too demanding. Do not concede too much by allowing objectives to be watered down to placate individuals. If you give in the practice will fail to meet its business objectives.

Hold this thought: be warned against setting unrealistic objectives, which will only produce a demoralised workforce and will be a breeding ground for feelings of inadequacy and resentment.

Human beings like to feel that their actions have a point to them (which is why objectives are important). If you do not set clear objectives, your employees may well do things themselves according to their own interpretation of what is required. Objectives are therefore important for learning and motivation. They are also your way of assessing how well everyone is working.

Rather than laying down (without discussion) the objectives for each employee, you should hold one-to-one meetings with them to discuss, negotiate, compromise and agree. Objectives may have to be a matter of meeting halfway, but you will at least then retain a willing and enthusiastic worker rather than turning them into someone who resents what you are trying to make them do.

Whenever you draw up a list of business objectives you will have to decide which ones are to come first and which ones can wait. Some may not even be achievable until earlier ones have been accomplished. Your list will need to reflect the importance of each objective and also set the timescale for the objectives as a whole.

Hold this thought: it is best to set a number of small, easily achievable personal objectives, rather than one bigger and not so achievable one.

The temptation is to think that because you are a dentist and your business is solely about doing dentistry, then that is all you have to do to be successful. It is important that as a business owner you devote some of your time to everything else around you that is going to contribute towards this success, that is, business planning.

Agree beforehand how performance will be measured

You must have a method or methods for measuring the progress being made towards the achievement of objectives, both personal and business. They must measure what is expected against how well the practice and its people are doing. You must keep methods simple and ensure that they are clearly understood by everyone.

Two words that you can use in your measurement systems are 'effective' and 'efficient'. These words are often incorrectly used, but the difference between them is simple: effective means doing the right thing and efficient means doing the thing right. You and your employees must be effective and efficient in everything you do.

Relate your performance measures to all aspects of the performance of the practice. Decide what to measure and why. Do not collect unnecessary information, only that which is relevant.

Measuring the success of individuals who have been set objectives related to increasing their knowledge is easy if there is an examination at the end. Other objectives may also be able to be measured in this way, but some may require an element of judgement. They may relate to how good/

accurate/relevant something was. Perhaps of more importance is the analysis of why objectives were *not* achieved. What got in the way?

You should develop the habit of setting objectives for almost everything you and your employees do. This is not over-managing or micro-managing, it is staying in control. Only by continuously doing this will you have a clear sense of direction and well-motivated employees who know exactly what is expected of them.

Objectives = appraisal

Keeping the practice on course depends upon everyone meeting his or her objectives. You should therefore carry out regular performance appraisals during which you can discuss with individuals how they are progressing. Past performance can be reviewed and new learning opportunities identified. The appraisal sessions give you and the appraisee the opportunity to set new objectives for the coming months and to revisit those already in place.

Appraisals are an excellent way of building a good rapport with your employees, provided you carry them out properly. For example, you must not:

- criticise employees on a personal level; always stick to how something relates to their work/performance
- avoid or dodge difficult issues; tackle thorny or contentious issues head on
- use closed questions; this will produce a monologue – you want a dialogue
- lose sight of the fact that change is unsettling, and that stretching an employee's potential can be threatening to them
- forget to praise good performance. Don't assume their achievements were easy. People always remember 'Thank you' and 'Well done'.

Hold this thought: if you have some bad news to deliver, begin with something positive, then give the bad news, then end on a positive note.

As the appraiser, you will hopefully:

- learn more about how each employee works
- understand their development, training and educational needs
- be able to motivate your employees
- improve communication.

Carried out properly, appraisals are a good way of motivating employees and are good for team building.

I used to appraise my employees at least once a year. The appraisal meetings enabled me to find out what made each employee tick. They were good for helping us all work more closely as a team. Patient care was therefore improved.

I remember one nurse who would never have won any prizes for her use of the English language, but she was an enthusiastic and willing worker who got on very well with the patients. I didn't dwell on her spelling mistakes or the way she sometimes used the wrong word; I focused more on her overall contribution to the success of the practice. This nurse was eventually poached by another practice.

(*See* 'Performance reviews (appraisal)' in Chapter 10 *Managing employees.*)

Taking your head out of the clouds

So far your mission statement and your objectives have been based on 'the ideal' – they represent your dream and are the things you would like to do if there were no restrictions. Now you have to come down to earth and weigh up the raw material that you have got to work with.

If you have so far succeeded in keeping your feet on the ground, what comes out of the next stage in the business planning process should not be too much of a shock, either to you or your employees.

Strengths (S), Weaknesses (W), Opportunities (O) and Threats (T)

SWOT is an acronym that crops up time and time again in a wide range of business activities. It can also apply on a personal level. (You should have carried it out on yourself when you were thinking of becoming a practice owner – *see* Section II.) People subconsciously carry out SWOT analyses on a range of activities, for example when looking for a new car or buying a new house, as well as for the smaller things in life. All you are doing in the context of your business is consciously going through the process in a more organised and structured fashion.

There are a number of key benefits to be gained from carrying out an *honest* SWOT analysis on your practice.

- It can provide the evidence for the need for (fundamental) change within the practice.
- It will help to uncover the core competencies of individuals and of the practice as a whole.
- It will help to secure the commitment and motivation (hopefully) of all of your employees.

The point has already been made that it is advisable to involve your employees when drawing up your practice mission statement and business objectives. For the same reasons, when assessing the strengths and weaknesses of the practice, you should also seek their opinions. If you exclude your employees, only part of the overall picture will emerge, and the missing pieces may be the ones that matter.

Again, it comes down to gathering information and then basing decisions on this information. Communicating these decisions to the rest of your employees and giving them the information on which the decisions are based helps to gain their agreement and cooperation.

Create a workshop environment and choose a leader or facilitator (this does not necessarily have to be you) who is able to encourage the free flow of thoughts and ideas. Set a timetable so that each component of the analysis receives equal time, as people will tend to spend too much time focusing on weaknesses.

Begin by examining the whole practice. The list of questions you could ask is endless, but to start off here are some of the main factors to think about:

- location
- access
- the building
- the décor
- the overall quality of the facilities
- the general quality of the treatment
- the level of training and development of the employees.

After work one day, first walk around the outside of the practice, then go inside, scrutinise every aspect of what you see. Imagine you are a potential patient. How might others see your practice?

What about the existing patients, are they loyal? (How is this measured?) What do they think about the practice? (How are you going to find out?)

Focus on the personal and professional strengths of the people within the practice.

- What are the strengths that are likely to give the practice a competitive edge in the future?
- What were the reasons for previous successes?

- What are the positive things that the employees contribute to the practice?
- How strong are the practice finances? It is no use having a grand plan that involves vast expenditure if the funds are simply not there.
- How strong is the overall management of the practice?

Embarking on an ambitious programme of change (which is what your business plan and strategy will inevitably involve) is going to require strong, professional management. Do you and/or your practice manager have these skills? Are you a strong enough leader?

> Strong management is something you must have in your business: either learn how to be an even better manager or buy in the skills by using an interim manager. I learnt how to do it myself, which took time, but it paid off in the end.

When discussing weaknesses, take care not to let the session become an opportunity for everyone to become involved in personally directed criticism. What is needed is an honest, objective appraisal of how things really are.

The questions you will need to answer are:

- Why has the practice not achieved the things you had hoped it would?
- What do you need to strengthen in order to succeed?
- Is there anything about the practice that puts people off?
- Who or what is the weak link in the chain?

You will need to remain very objective when talking to your employees about all of this. You will naturally feel protective about what is after all your business, perhaps something you started from scratch.

Hold this thought: Aristophanes' cloud cuckoo land is the last place you want to be.

The majority of weaknesses in any organisation are usually 'people' problems. Your practice will be no different.

> My wife and I used to do a bit of practice management consultancy. It was amazing how many of the problems in practices stemmed from the owner. Part of the problem is that practice owners are often blinkered to their own weaknesses and are extremely unwilling to even consider the need to change or modify their behaviour.

Strengths and weaknesses tend to be internal factors, whereas opportunities and threats are more to do with external factors. To help you come up with a list of external factors apply the acronym STEP, that is, things that come under the headings of social, technological, economic and political.

Thinking carefully about the opportunities that may exist in the future should eventually suggest the way forward. Inevitably, this part of the business planning process must involve the appraisal of every aspect of the practice and a detailed exploration of what currently might be considered to be weaknesses and threats, but which you hope to turn into winning opportunities.

This section of the SWOT analysis provides the practice with the reasons for introducing new products or services and for assessing the benefits they might bring. You must be prepared to challenge the status quo and to look for very good reasons for remaining exactly as you are at present.

Remember that the opportunities that exist today may not be there tomorrow, and may actually be tomorrow's threats, so decide whether you need to act quickly, or whether you can afford to let them slip by and wait for better ones to turn up later.

Threats are obviously the opposite of opportunities. Failure to seize your opportunities as they arise may mean that they later become threats. Set up a worst-case scenario, but do not be too pessimistic. The fact that you are thinking about the threats to your business probably means that you will do something to limit their effect.

Challenges, not problems

You should neither get carried away into believing that nothing about the practice has to change, nor should you become too depressed because you think that everything about it is wrong. If you have set your sights too high you will have a mountain to climb, but that does not mean that you cannot do it.

Build on the strengths and look forward to the opportunities. Regard the elimination of weaknesses and threats as a challenge, not as an insurmountable problem.

Your list of ideas, suggestions and possible recommendations that have been compiled from the SWOT analysis must be fed back into your objectives. Your objectives should determine which are the key elements of the SWOT analysis that will demand (urgent) attention. You must concentrate on the most important and relevant elements. Stay focused!

> Business ownership can sometimes be a lonely place, leaving you with the feeling that no one else is going through what you are going through. I was lucky because I did have someone to talk to, someone who fully understood and appreciated the nightmare that running your own business can sometimes be. However, you need not feel on your own: there are groups out there that help to bring together practice owners and managers so they can discuss the day-to-day problems everyone has. You should never feel that you have to cope with problems on your own. You could always start your own group.

13

Strategic planning

When one door closes, another opens; but we often look so long and so regrettably upon the closed door that we do not see the one which has opened for us.

(Alexander Graham Bell)

This chapter is going to show you how to formulate the long-term strategic plan that is going to help you build a successful practice. Perhaps a more apposite term might be 'stratagem', that is, 'a plan or scheme intended to outwit an opponent'. If you simply follow the herd you will end up where every one else ends up; but if you are one step ahead of the game you can gain a significant competitive business advantage over other practices.

The word 'strategy' is derived from the Greek *strategia* which means leader or general in charge of an army. Nowadays a strategy refers to a high level plan to achieve one or more goals, usually under conditions of uncertainty. Isn't this the background against which a dental practice usually operates?

If your mission statement represents the general direction in which you want to head and your objectives more specifically where you are heading for, your strategy sets out how you intend to get there. However, one of the problems with strategic planning is that it all too often becomes an exercise in simply repeating what happened last year. Strategy is the thing that drives the practice forward, helping it achieve its objectives, and which is concerned with long-term planning – a period of between 2 and 5 years. Short-term factors are usually dealt with in your business plan.

Hold this thought: the challenge is to look at things in a totally new way, to identify new markets, new products or methods of working, which are going to give the practice an advantage over its competitors.

Strategic planning goes right to the heart of the practice and the business. It asks key questions.

- Where is the practice now?
- How did it get there?
- What business is it in?
- Where does it want to be in the future?
- How is it going to get there?

Even if you are relatively happy with where the practice is now, it is still a worthwhile exercise revisiting how it got there. Are there any lessons to be learnt?

Without strategic planning you will lack the framework that can enable the practice to:

- understand its position within the current marketplace. Do you even know what the current marketplace is?
- move forward with a sense of direction, purpose and urgency. Lack of direction and purpose, and inertia stifles any business
- focus on quality, patients and productivity
- improve the motivation of the employees
- change to bring about all round improvement.

Failure to plan will mean that the practice will always have to react to situations; it will always be vulnerable to threats and will most likely miss opportunities.

Every now and again I used to take myself well away from the practice and, armed only with a blank piece of paper and a pen, let my mind wander into all sorts of thoughts, ideas and concepts about how to improve the practice. I didn't want to make changes for change's sake, but I wanted to explore the seemingly impossible.

A few years after I gave up clinical dentistry I gave a talk to a dental audience about the first edition of this book. At the end one of the delegates, a dentist who worked near to where I had worked but whom I had never met, announced that I had always been one step ahead of other dentists in my thinking about practice management. I didn't think I was doing anything different, but clearly I was.

Answering the difficult questions

1. Where is the practice now?

You need to analyse the recent performance of the practice in relation to the market, both locally and regionally, and in relation to the industry as a whole.

- Can you find out how the performance of your practice compares to others in the industry? What is your market share? NASDAL accountants should have all of this statistical information you need to answer these questions.
- What do your patients think of you and the practice? You must find out whether or not you are satisfying (or exceeding) your patients' expectations.
- What are the *real* strengths (and weaknesses) of the practice that makes the difference between you and the competition?
- Do you know if the practice is growing, stagnant or declining? If so, how is this being measured? Are you looking at this in terms of number of patients, number of new patients, turnover, or profit?

2. How did it get there?

Wherever you are now, whether or not it is where you want to be, it is important to assess the reasons and factors that combined to create the current situation.

- What has the practice done right (or wrong) to get there?
- What has it done well (or badly)?
- Was the practice just in the right place at the right time?
- Is the practice here because of good planning, bad planning or no planning at all?

3. What business is it in?

This may seem an absurd question (it is a dental practice!) but what you do goes a lot deeper than that. You are a service industry competing with other service industries (ask your patients how often they go to the hairdresser and how much they spend each time) as well as leisure industries (how many will happily pay relatively high fees to join a health club, but will still insist on having the cheapest treatment they can?). Many dental practices now offer a wider range of services, other than just dentistry, including Botox, that all come under the banner of 'cosmetic' treatment'.

4. Where does it want to be in the future?

Are you going to be a general practice or are you going to specialise? Are you going to branch out and offer a wider range of cosmetic treatments? Are you going to miss out on opportunities if you limit the scope of the practice, or is specialisation going to allow you to tap into a more enjoyable and rewarding niche market?

You must think long and hard about what are the core strengths of the practice and then build on them. Do not fall into the trap of discarding what you may have spent years putting together just because something else seems more attractive. This does not mean that you cannot change the practice, but always work from your strengths rather than starting from some point that may be weaker.

> A friend of mine, a management consultant at KPMG, uses a lovely phrase to describe businesses that have diversified and have as a consequence taken their eye off their core business, which suffered as a result. He calls it 'diworseification'. Bear this is mind before you diversify.

5. How is it going to get there?

In deciding where you want to be in the future you will be building on your strengths. Conversely, when you are deciding how you are going to get there you will have to concentrate on eliminating your weaknesses. The focus is on the elimination of anything that might inhibit progress.

Examine factors such as:

- the changes that are likely to take place in the market
- the changes in patients' attitudes and expectations
- the improvements in technology
- what your competitors are doing.

Then consider internal factors, which will include:

- training and development of employees
- improving the services on offer
- the overall performance of the practice
- how success is going to be measured
- how the proposed improvements are going to be funded.

Well thought out and planned strategies do not come to fruition overnight. You need to set realistic timeframes that take into account the complexity of the task and the resources required.

Your strategy should take you through a 5-year period, within which you should have prioritised items and calculated how long each of those items will take to complete. You should double your estimate of the length of time any task is likely to take.

Your strategic plan should not be set in stone. Don't put your practice in a straitjacket. If it is, the practice will not be able to respond to sudden changes; it will not be responsive to changing market conditions.

Hold this thought: your strategic plan must be creative and challenging, but above all it should be focused.

You may have to go back and review your objectives once you have formulated your strategies. You may never be able to achieve 'perfect' objectives or a 'perfect' strategy; perhaps the most you can hope for at any one time is a 'best fit'.

Problems with strategic planning

Like most other things in life, strategic planning comes with its own set of potential problems. You and your employees might be ready to implement your strategy, but you find that nothing or very little happens. Why? Strategic planning can fail to deliver for a number of reasons.

- One person (you?) dominates the process and fails to take account of the views of your employees and patients.
- Complacency – you and your employees are not convinced that things need to be changed.
- Change is brought about for its own sake with no consideration for the consequences.
- Objective setting is rushed and goals are too vague.

- Strategies are not fully developed because of time-pressures (real or imaginary).
- You do not remain fully committed to what is being proposed.
- You do not believe in the process of 'planning' and therefore want to see it fail.
- The practice is so close to going bust that no amount of strategic planning will help.

Taking each one of these problems in turn:

- you have dominated the process because you know best, or so you think
- you are happy to continue drifting along as you are
- you think you have to change but fail to think through the knock-on effects
- you rush at the whole business and strategic planning process without thinking things through properly
- nothing seems to happen at first so you lose interest and boredom sets in
- you thought you'd give 'management' a go, but as you don't believe in it (I'm a dentist, not a manager) your heart's not in it
- perhaps you've left it all too late?

To remain ahead of your competitors you must constantly scan the social, technological, economic and political (STEP) environment. Your business does not exist in isolation. Your customers respond in the same way as everyone else's do to social changes, advances in technology, rises in mortgage rates or a change of government. Each one of these will have an impact on your practice whether you like it or not.

You should read the business section of newspapers to find out what is going on in the wider business world. Speculation about interest and mortgage rate rises will dampen consumer demand for products and services.

Find out what is going on in the local economy by talking to your patients about their work. Find out whether a large employer in the area is expanding or laying off workers. Are there any new commercial or housing developments in the pipeline?

Your practice manager should have been doing all of this already.

> I enjoyed talking to my patients and finding out where they worked and what they did for a job. People who were in business for themselves shared their experiences with me. I learnt a great deal.

Every business decision you make carries some element of risk. When you are formulating your strategic plan you must always build in a risk limitation factor and have contingency plans that minimise the impact of any adverse event. Always try to quantify the risk element of any proposal and then consider the risk–benefit implications. Don't think that by simply doing nothing you will eliminate business risk: standing still leaves you vulnerable to being left behind or, worse still, being crushed in the rush as other practices steam ahead into new markets.

Don't forget that you must also have insurance to cover major losses or disruption to your business. Permanent health insurance for you and for any equity partners is also very important.

> I speak from personal experience when I say that you must have permanent health insurance (PHI). I had to take out life insurance when I bought a house and when I bought my practice, but no one ever suggested that I might need PHI in case I didn't die but was unable to work. I took it upon myself to take out PHI and I am glad I did.

Most dentists are good at drawing up treatment plans, but mention strategic planning to them and their eyes glaze over as if you've suddenly started to speak a foreign language. However, if you stop for a moment and think about the two processes you'll see that there are many similarities, and therefore being able to draw up a strategic plan is something a dentist should be well equipped to do.

A treatment plan begins with a patient's dental history, which should be a chronological account of what has happened or not happened to them in the past dental wise. In other words, what has brought the patient to the point they are at now? A dental history poses the same two questions as do the first two questions in the strategic planning process, namely, 'Where is the practice/business now?' And 'How did it get there?'

You take and record a patient's medical history, which in many respects is similar to working out at an early stage what are going to be the limiting factors that will affect your treatment plan. I'll come to limiting factors in the strategic planning process later.

Then comes the examination, during which you see for yourself what you've actually got to work with or perhaps more importantly, what you *haven't* got! You might need to carry out some 'special tests', for example, radiographs, a full periodontal assessment, vitality tests, or obtain study models for occlusal analysis. You might need to consult with specialists or seek a second opinion. You are carrying out a subconscious SWOT analysis of the patient's dental health, which is exactly what you would do in the strategic planning process after you have tackled the first two strategic planning questions. Overriding all of this might be the patient's medical history that, perhaps because of one or more factors, is going to limit what you can do or achieve for them.

One of the questions that strategic planning throws up and the one that seems to cause the most head scratching is, 'What business is the practice in?' On a much simpler level, though, the question is asking what type of dentistry do you offer, is it general, specialist or (the latest term) cosmetic? This is the opportunities and threats you uncovered as part of your SWOT analysis. It is the same with your treatment planning; do you want to offer only simple treatment options or are you going to offer a specialised, highly technical option.

The diagnosis is the next step. Here you set out what is wrong, before making recommendations as to how you propose to put things right. This is not dissimilar to the next strategic planning question, 'Where does the practice/business want to be in the future?' For both processes you will be thinking about the 'ideal', but you know there are likely to be things that are going to prevent or inhibit progress towards your goal. In terms of your dental treatment plan, it might be the patient's attitude towards dentistry or their financial situation. Strategically, it might be that one or more members of your team are underperforming; you may feel that your practice premises need to be modernised or that the practice is in the wrong place for the type of business you want to run. But as with your patient, it might all come down to the availability of money.

The building blocks that will underpin your actual treatment plan are now all in place. The treatment plan itself falls into three phases: short, medium, and long term. This is the same as the next strategic planning question, 'How is the practice/business going to get to where it wants to be?' Your short-term treatment plan addresses the pressing issues, such as relief of pain and sepsis, as well as the beginnings of the restoration of function and aesthetics. Your immediate thoughts for your strategic plan might be deciding what or who has to go or change or improve, and what or who can stay. This again brings you back to the strengths and weaknesses in your SWOT analysis. Your medium- and long-term treatment plans are aimed at stabilisation, improvement and, if necessary, changing the attitude of the patient so that they see the benefits of what you are doing for them and so are more willing to accept more advanced (and costlier) treatment. This is what your medium- and longer-term strategic plans also hope to achieve: stabilisation of the business in terms of its finance, its employees and its patient base, followed by all round improvement in every aspect of the practice.

I'm sorry if some of the connections between treatment planning and strategic planning might at times seem a bit tenuous, but overall I hope it makes sense to you. If you think of strategic planning as 'A plan of action to achieve a desired goal', this could equally be applied to your treatment plans. I have often said that any final treatment plan evolves out of trying to draw the patient closer and closer to what you as a professional are recommending. So too your strategic plan often ends up as being a 'best fit' rather than the 'ideal'.

Hold this thought: trying to manage your business without having a mission statement, objectives, strategies, a business plan or budgets is a bit like trying to do a full mouth rehabilitation without a treatment plan!

Pulling everything together: your business plan

It is now time to start pulling everything together and begin writing your business plan. Your practice manager should be able to help you make a start with this; however, you may not want to leave it entirely up to them to produce the finished document. It is your business and it is therefore your plan.

You began the business planning process by considering your mission. You then moved on to set your objectives, and finally you formulated your strategy. Your business plan, with the addition of financial information, is the end result of this process. A business plan is therefore an essential document for your practice, being as it is a written summary of what you hope to accomplish by being in business, and how you intend to organise your resources to meet your objectives. It must contain the mission, objectives and strategy of the practice but, most importantly, it enables you to measure progress towards their achievement.

You should not even attempt to write your business plan until everything that has previously been set out in this section has been completed. The message again is take your time, don't move on to the next thing until you've have the previous thing absolutely right.

You should refresh your memory about what a finished business plan looks like by going back to Section II *Purchase*.

Hold this thought: the success of any business plan depends a great deal on the clarity and realism of the thought behind it, its comprehensiveness and how well it is put together.

Review what you have already discovered

The SWOT analysis will have provided you with much of the evidence for the changes that are needed if you are to achieve your business objectives. Before you commit yourself to paper review what the SWOT analysis is telling you. Does it all add up? Are you sure that what you propose follows on from what you have discovered? This is an invaluable exercise. Remember that the business plan is mainly for your benefit, but that it might also be read by others, for example, your bank manager, so you must be honest and realistic in your assessment of your proposals. You may have to convince others that you have thoroughly researched the market, that you have anticipated problems, and that you have thought about how you are going to overcome them.

The basic format

A business plan describes three elements of your practice, namely:

- operations: the premises in which the practice is located; equipment; employees; the services on offer
- finance: set-up costs (if it is a new practice or a new surgery within an existing practice); fixed and variable costs once the practice/surgery is up and running; minimal financial requirements
- marketing: how potential customers are going to be approached.

There are a number of sections to a business plan and they are all equally important.

1. Set the scene.
    - Give a brief description of yourself: your clinical experience, your management experience, and your personal goals. A well-written curriculum vitae is extremely useful.
    - Describe who your customers are: where they are from, their social class and age distribution.
    - Include any key factors that may affect the success of the practice.
2. Set out your objectives.
    - List short-term targets that together make up your longer term objectives.
    - Set out a series of short steps that are achievable and measurable.

3. Set out your analysis of the market – the overall market and that part of it you are going to target. You will need to include:
   - details of your proposed customers
   - who your competitors will be
   - sources of alternative services for your customers
   - any other factors that might influence the market.
4. Set out your approach to marketing your services.
   - What image does your practice wants to project?
   - Describe the promotional material that you are going to use. Include examples in an appendix.
   - What is unique about your practice that will differentiate it from others?
   - Set out your assessment of the four 'Ps' of the marketing mix: product, price, place, promotion. (Some marketing people include a fifth 'P', people.)
5. Describe your future plans for researching and developing your services.
6. Set out your financial plan (this will be of most interest to any lending source).
   - What are the start-up costs going to be for any proposed expansion?
   - Include a cash-flow projection for next year's trading.
   - Include a detailed budget for the coming year and a rough guide for the following year.
   - Include an accurate breakeven projection.

   You will have to show any lender that tight control of incoming and outgoing funds is in place. You should always bear in mind that it is not profitability that decides whether or not you will stay in business; it is cash flow. Details of how to draw up a budget and a cash-flow forecast are discussed later in this section.
7. Give an accurate appraisal of the strength of the management of the practice. A well-managed business is less likely to experience difficulties because any difficulties are more likely to be anticipated and dealt with correctly. If you have no management experience, say so, but say where your management advice is going to come from. This will impress any potential lender.
8. Highlight any risks and problems that you have identified. Show that you have thought carefully about these and indicate how you propose to deal with them.
9. Finish your plan with your main conclusions, making sure that you leave the reader with a very positive impression. Include key features, such as:
   - your strategic plan
   - the strengths of the practice
   - the unique selling points of the practice
   - realistic income and expenditure projections.
10. Your plan should include an executive summary that, although mentioned last, actually appears at the beginning. It is a complete, overall summary of every part of the plan.

You must not be too optimistic with your plan. Don't assume that the reader is going to be swept along by your enthusiasm: you will have to convince some cynics.

Writing a good business plan takes time. You should, if necessary, seek help from people with the relevant experience and knowledge and, most importantly, you should be prepared to listen to them.

Set out the plan logically and make sure that it is well written. Simplify, but don't oversimplify; draft and redraft until it is right. If you are writing your plan because you are about to buy your first practice, or because you are planning to expand an existing practice, or because you are experiencing difficulties with your existing practice, the plan might be your first step on the road to success.

Hold this thought: you will have less difficulty convincing anyone of the viability of your proposal if you have taken the time and trouble to critically analyse every stage.

(*See* 'The practice manager as business manager' in Chapter 12 *Business planning.*)

What use is your business plan once you have written it?

If you have diligently followed the process of business planning from start to finish, you will by now have invested a great deal of time and effort in the process. You must not therefore allow your business plan to gather dust on a shelf or to be consigned to some never-opened filing cabinet. It is a working document that you should refer to frequently, certainly at least once every 3 months (more often is not a bad thing) when you update your cash-flow forecast.

You must check to see whether what you have predicted has actually happened and, if it has not, then what has gone wrong? Ask yourself, 'What do I need to do to get the practice back on track?' Make your business plan work for you through it being there as a constant reminder of the things you hope to achieve. It should provide motivation.

Spending 15–30 minutes at the end of each month to review and revise (remember, your plan is not set in stone) your business plan is time well spent.

Once I had written my business plan I used to review it at the end of every month. If it looked like the practice was veering off course I would take swift action to get it back on track.

When I wanted to change banks I could present a professional-looking business plan to them, which I am sure helped me in my negotiations.

14

Financial planning

It was Mr Micawber in *David Copperfield* who uttered the immortal words:

Annual income twenty pounds, annual expenditure nineteen pounds nineteen and six, result happiness. Annual income twenty pounds, annual expenditure twenty pounds nought and six, result misery.

Annual budgets and cash-flow projections

This subsection deals with drawing up a budget and a cash-flow projection for the coming 12 months.

Budgeting is central to how you will measure the success of your strategic plan. It is obviously also an essential tool for monitoring the financial progress of the practice.

Hold this thought: budgets and cash-flow projections are a vital defence against bankruptcy.

You should draw up your annual budget and cash-flow projection not less than 3 months prior to the start of the year (calendar or financial). It goes without saying that your projection for the coming year should be more accurate than those for years two, three, four and five.

There are a number of other advantages to having a budget.

- It is an effective way of allocating funds.
- It gives you a method of communicating important financial information to others, both inside and outside the practice.
- It helps you to think about and visualise the financial implications of your future plans.
- It provides a method of measuring the performance of everyone in the practice.
- The bottom line is that it gives you greater control of your business.

Budgeting can only be undertaken when you have clearly defined your objectives and set out your strategic plan. Objectives and strategic plans always have a financial dimension, so build their costs into your budget and cash-flow projections.

Hold this thought: until you know what you want to do you cannot possibly begin to make an estimate of the likely cost.

Medium- and long-term financial planning

Your medium- and long-term strategic plans need to be expressed in financial terms. You must therefore draw up a rough (but accurate) budget and cash-flow projection to cover this period. You may think it is going to be difficult to predict these figures with any great accuracy, but you should nevertheless try to build up a picture.

Annual budgets have already been dealt with earlier in this chapter, but looking further ahead, you should always also consider the longer term financial management of the practice.

- Are you going to need finance for the purchase of premises, equipment etc?
- What is the trend likely to be with regard to your turnover?
- What is going to happen to your costs?

Your prediction for year two should be more accurate than for year three and so on, but by carrying out this exercise you will get a feel for how the practice finances are going to look over the longer term.

Hold this thought: think about your strategic plan; is it a plan for growth, stagnation or regression?

> As I have said, trying to manage your practice without having objectives, strategies, a business plan or budgets is a bit like trying to do a full mouth rehabilitation without a treatment plan. Trying to manage your business without any regard for finance is impossible.
>
> Once I had taken my practice through the whole business planning process I felt as if I was at last in control of my business. A great deal of the uncertainty and unpredictability, which had been there for some time, suddenly disappeared.

Drawing up your budget

You should by now have an accurate annual budget; you now have to break it down into monthly chunks. This enables you to manage the budget as the year progresses, to spot variances and to take early, effective, corrective action. Begin by setting out your budget figures for each month, and then as the year progresses enter the 'real' figures in the income and expenditure columns.

You need to understand how to operate a budget sheet and the importance of certain elements within it.

1. Opening balance – to give as true a picture as possible you should use the balance in your cashbook. If you don't use a cashbook I suggest you start using one now! A negative (overdrawn) figure is always shown in brackets.

2. Income – self-explanatory, but is it going to vary from one month to the next?

3. Fixed costs – these are the costs that have to be met whether or not you carry out any treatment, or even if the door to the practice remains shut.

4. Breakeven point – this is a critical figure and one that you must know if you are to control your budget and cash flow during the year. Your breakeven point represents the income you need to generate in order to cover your fixed costs, that is, the costs associated with just being open, let alone carrying out any treatments. This is a 'working' definition that does not include an element of variable costs and marginal costing theory. Your breakeven point should not vary significantly from one month to the next. The significance of breakeven point is obvious. If over a period of months you are unable to pay your fixed costs you are heading for financial meltdown.

5. Variable costs – these are costs whose size depends on the amount of work you do and are related to laboratory costs, materials etc.

6. Drawings – this is what you draw from the business for your personal use.

7. Cash flow in (out) – this is calculated using the formula: Income minus Fixed costs minus Variable costs minus Drawings.

8. Closing balance – this is the opening balance plus or minus (depending on whether the cash flow was positive or negative) the cash-flow figure. The closing balance from one month is carried forward to the next month, where it now becomes the opening balance.

Hold this thought: you must always aim to keep your breakeven point as low as possible.

Controlling your budget

The main benefit of drawing up a budget is that it gives you the means of monitoring (and controlling) practice expenditure. If you fail to control your budget:

Budget and Cash flow projection for year beginning: _____

| | January | | February | | March | | April | | May | | June | | July | | August | | September | | October | | November | | December | | Total | |
	Budget	Actual	Budget	Actual	Budget	Actual	Budget	Actual	Budget	Actual	Budget	Actual	Budget	Actual	Budget	Actual	Budget	Actual	Budget	Actual	Budget	Actual	Budget	Actual	Budget	Actual
Opening balance																										
Income																										
Fixed costs																										
Breakeven																										
Variable costs																										
Drawings																										
Cash flow In (Out)																										
Closing balance																										

Figure 14.1 Budget and cash-flow projection

- you may frequently overspend and so run into difficulties with your bank
- you will lack up-to-date financial information, which may be required urgently by third parties, for example, your bank
- It demonstrates your lack of control of the business as a whole.

You should develop the habit of gathering information, and not just financial, as near to the event as possible; within 3 working days of the month-end is not unreasonable.

Hold this thought: it is always preferable to have almost accurate information on time rather than accurate information late.

Controlling your budget is therefore very important and once you have mastered the technique it is relatively straightforward.

You should ensure that you:

- understand the figures. You must take the time to familiarise yourself with each one and understand its significance
- decide how often you are going to monitor the budget. As a rule of thumb, the more perilous your financial position, the more frequently you need to (must!) look at the figures
- have an early warning system. This could be when your income falls below a certain level or when your costs rise over a given period
- quickly identify variances
- talk with those who help you stick to the budget; don't suffer in silence
- act quickly to get the budget back on course. You could do nothing (thinking that it is just a blip), revise your budget or take firm corrective action
- continuously monitor the budget.

You must not:

- make decisions to correct your budget based on knee-jerk reactions
- try to go it alone by not discussing the problem with your employees. It is not an admission of failure if you ask for their help
- try to ignore the problem; it will definitely not go away!

> I monitored my budget and cash flow very carefully. I was not going to wait until my bank statement dropped through the letterbox at the end of the month before I knew the state of my bank balance.

Cash flow in more detail

Your practice may generate a profit, but the level of profit may not accurately reflect the financial health (and viability) of the business. Unless cash can be generated throughout the year to pay wages this week, next week and every other week, then soon there will be no more weeks. Your practice must always have the funds on hand to pay its bills as they fall due for payment. A negative cash flow, even for a profitable practice, will ultimately lead to its demise. This might be a stark message, but it is reality.

Hold this thought: it is critical that you understand the difference between profit and cash flow.

While controlling a budget is nearly always a retrospective exercise, controlling cash flow is very much about forward planning. You should regard cash flow as something dynamic and as something that can change (very) rapidly. Even if you generate a profit there may still be periods during the year when you may not have the money to pay your bills. By monitoring the net inflow (and outflow) of funds into (and out of) your account, and by looking ahead to your immediate future financial commitments, you should know when you would be best able to settle outstanding bills.

Hold this thought: delaying payment in the face of mounting bills does not improve your cash flow; it merely puts off the inevitable (usually to a time when you will be less able to pay).

Controlling cash flow is important because it will:

- tell you where your cash is tied up
- allow you to spot in advance potential periods of cash starvation
- reduce your dependency on your bank. A bank manager has been described as someone who will lend you an umbrella when the sun is shining, but will want it back when it starts to rain; do not let your bank control your business
- give you greater control of your business.

There are several areas of your practice in which cash may be unnecessarily tied up.

1. Material stock
   - Are you holding more stock than is absolutely necessary?
   - Have you bought materials in greater quantities because of bulk discount offers and in so doing so tied up money that could (should) have been used for other, more necessary purchases?
   - Do you have a stock control system in place and, if so, is it working? If you do not have one, you need one.
   - Who is responsible for ordering? Is there a budget in operation and who controls it?
2. Credit control
   - Debtors are people or companies that owe you money (they are in debt to you). If your debtors delay payment, it follows that you may in turn be unable to pay your bills. You must squeeze your debtors to reduce the pressure they exert on the smooth financial management of your practice. This can be achieved by:
     1. collecting patient payments as near to the start of treatment as possible
     2. monitoring and controlling the amount of money sitting in your current file
     3. adopting a very strict debt collection policy.
   - Creditors are people and companies that you owe money to (they have given you credit). Most companies allow up to 30 days or a month's credit. You should use this period. However, if you do not make payment within this time, as time passes, creditors become increasingly more demanding for payment. Most practices have creditors ranging from a few hundred pounds to several thousands. However, it is not just the size of the debt that can cause you sleepless nights, it is also the age of the debt, bearing in mind the older the debt, the greater the urgency on the part of the creditor for settlement.
   - Creditors will take legal action to recover their money; do not ignore their demands for payment. Pre-empt legal action by agreeing a repayment schedule long before it reaches that stage. If need be you should approach your creditors and negotiate an extension to your credit period, as long as it does not involve any excessive penalty interest costs.
3. Cash tied up in fixed assets
   - Have you tied money up unnecessarily in fixed assets?
   - Could assets be leased rather than purchased with cash?
   - Are the assets used or could they be disposed of?
   - Have you invested in assets that could be replaced by something a little more modest?
   - Has money been invested for vanity rather than for profit?

Do you know how much potential income is sitting in your current file? One practice I worked in was obviously having cash-flow problems because the owner was constantly telling his associates to spend time going through their current file, and getting patients in to complete treatment, send bills to those who had not returned, and get any NHS forms off to the Board. Clearing out your current file should give your cash flow a sudden shot in the arm.

Month	Jan	Feb	March	April	May	June	July	August	Sept
Company name									
Company A	£	££							
Company B	£	0							
Company C	£	££							
Company D	£	£							
Company E	£	£							
Total owed this month	£££££	££££££							

Figure 14.2 Quick cash-flow chart

To help you visualise your cash flow, use a time chart to monitor and anticipate potential cash-flow problems. This is easy to do, and seeing it all set out will make you aware of your spending habits.

To draw up this chart list every company/supplier/laboratory you deal with down the left hand column, and across the top of the page write the months. Whenever you buy anything on credit, receive an invoice, or a monthly statement, list it against the company/supplier/laboratory's name and enter the amount to be paid in the vertical column for the month it falls due. You will quickly build up a picture of exactly how much and when these bills have to be settled. If you do not settle a particular bill in any particular month, move the debt to the right, to the next month. Seeing your liabilities set out like this helps you to see in which months you might have trouble meeting your variable costs.

In this example, the amounts owed to Companies A and C in January were still outstanding in February, but more goods or services had been bought from them. The outstanding amount to Company A had risen, as had the amount owed to Company C. Only Company B had been paid at the end of January. Companies D and E's bills had also not been settled in January, although for now the amount owing had not increased. The total amount owed to all creditors has risen between January and February, and Companies A and C are more likely to start pressing for payment than they were at the end of January. If this pattern of ordering and non-payment were to continue throughout the year, not only would the amount owing have increased, but several companies would be pressing for payment.

Hold this thought: if your creditors (and this includes your bank) have got you over a barrel, your aim should be to get as far away from the barrel as possible.

Stock control

Controlling stock is about deciding what, when and how much to order. It is also about controlling money.

The first stage is to set a budget, which can be monthly, quarterly or annually based. The budget must be monitored, so appoint someone whose responsibility it is. Then you need a stock controller whose job it is to replenish stock.

Dental materials are expensive. They were when I gave up clinical dentistry and I don't suppose they are any cheaper now. When you look at a box of restorative material, don't see it as that, see it as pound notes sitting in your store room. The more stock you hold, the more of your money is tied up and therefore the less money you have to spend on other, perhaps more urgent, things.

Retailers have got stock control off to a fine art; after all they don't want tens of thousands of pounds sitting around. Most of these businesses operate what is known as 'just in time' stock control, where they order new stock so that it arrives as near to when it is needed as possible. For this to work they have to know their suppliers' lead-in times. For food retailers 'Use by dates' are critical: unsold products have to be disposed of, usually with no or little cash return. In dentistry, out-of-date materials represent waste.

How can you implement an effective stock control system so that you never run out of things, while at the same time never carry any out-of-date stock?

- Identify the materials you use the most (the ones with the highest turnover).
- Identify the materials you need, but which you use infrequently (the ones that are most likely to run out of date).
- Review the last 6 months' orders to work out how long each item took to arrive from the time it was ordered. This represents your lead-in time.
- Review how frequently each item was ordered. This plus the lead-in times are key factors in your stock control system.
- Put together a full stock list showing the lead-in time of every item.

Once your system is up and running, the next things you must do are:

- review current stock levels, and use up anything that is close to its use by date
- pull anything that is about to expire to the front – practise 'First in, first out'
- when you receive an order, check that not only is it what you ordered, but that it also has a sufficient shelf life – if it hasn't, send it back

By adopting a methodical approach to stock control you should:

- hold minimum stock levels, thereby not tying money up
- never have anything that has to be thrown out because it has passed its expiry date
- hopefully, stay within budget.

In the background, you should always maintain accurate records of what has been ordered and from where.

My wife exercises a very strict stock control regime in our kitchen. We shop, and like every other household we accumulate spices, ingredients, jams, pickles, sauces etc., some of which are used once or twice then get pushed to the back of the cupboard. Once, say, every 3 months she pulls everything out, checks the use-by dates and either throws things out, or works out how to use up the short shelf life stuff before it exceeds its use by date. Very little is wasted.

Preserving current profit levels

Tight budgetary control is a very effective way of preserving your current profit levels at times of decreasing income, and of increasing profit during times of stagnation. If your income is falling there is only one way to protect your profit and that is to cut your costs.

Periods of negative cash flow can be countered by reducing costs, which is a much more immediate and effective method of rectification than trying to increase your income, which usually takes a lot longer.

Hold this thought: aggressively reducing costs is something you must be prepared to do.

Going up, standing still or cutting back?

Almost every practice aims (hopes) to expand; it supposedly brings financial security.

Your aims with any expansion programme should be to:

- increase your turnover
- increase your profit
- improve your cash flow.

How to expand a practice is dealt with in more detail later in this chapter, but for now, whenever you are planning to expand you must always work through the likely cash-flow implications very carefully beforehand. You will be hoping for an improvement in your profit, but if your cash-flow situation deteriorates as a consequence, as it often can if the expansion is not carefully managed, you may not remain in business long enough to enjoy the fruits of your labours.

Hold this thought: your budget and cash-flow projections for a period of planned growth (the emphasis is on planned) must always be very carefully thought through.

Remaining as you are, at least for the time being, should not always be thought of as a backward step. If your analysis of the current position of the practice and the current market is such that change is undesirable, plan accordingly. You should, however, try to limit any increase in costs, at least until you are absolutely sure which way things are moving, to protect or slightly increase your profit.

Cutting back may sometimes be an option that on the face of it is unthinkable, but which might in the short term be the way forward. The importance of cash flow (as opposed to profitability) has already been stressed, but recognising when and knowing how to close loss-making gaps could save your practice from financial ruin. Forcefully cutting costs while allowing your turnover to fall can turn a negative cash-flow situation into a positive one. Going for an increase in turnover with the associated increase in costs could only hasten the very thing you are trying to escape from, that is, a loss-making and/or negative cash-flow situation.

> Dentists don't go into dentistry to be accountants, but you cannot neglect the importance of the financial management of your practice. In my early days as a practice owner I was blasé about money; I'd come from being an associate in a practice where there was more work and consequently more money than I knew what to do with. I learnt the hard way once money had to be managed. You should, rather than simply letting your accountant hand you your profit and loss account and a fat bill at the end of each year, ask them to go through and explain every heading so that you at least have some understanding of what it all means. However, one thing the profit and loss accounts don't show, and which is probably more important, is cash flow. That is your province.

Planning for additional profit

Squeezing greater profit out of your practice is something that can be achieved without compromising clinical standards and/or customer care, but only if you and your team all work more effectively and efficiently. There are several ways in which greater profit can be generated.

- Increase the amount of treatment you do.
- Reduce costs.
- Recover costs where this had previously not been the case.
- Change the product mix.
- Selectively raise prices.
- Reduce the capital invested in the practice.

The above are all interrelated: changes to one will affect others. However, changes do not necessarily always have the desired effect on your profit.

Hold this thought: you are more likely to see your profit rise if instead of focusing on the above you concentrate on improving your customer care.

An excellent customer care programme helps to keep your patients happy, and it motivates your employees.

> I would prefer to have a practice that gives excellent care to all its patients, has happy staff, of course happy patients, low overheads, a very low breakeven point, and a profit that I don't have to kill myself to achieve, rather than one that has the biggest turnover in the country, but which is a nightmare to work in.

Consider your costs

Before you go any further, ask yourself, 'Do I actually know how much it costs to run my surgery, and the other surgeries in my practice, per month, per week, per hour?' If you don't know perhaps you need to find out.

Your costs fall broadly into two groups: fixed and variable. Fixed costs are those that happen anyway, while variable costs only happen when you carry out treatment, and they generally rise the more treatment you do.

Divide your anticipated costs under whatever headings best suit your circumstances. Look at last year's budget (if you had one) or your profit and loss accounts, and use those headings as a starting point.

Estimate the amount you will spend per item per month. You will have to make assumptions, but with a little effort you can make your estimates as accurate as possible. Remember to include items that do not occur monthly, but perhaps quarterly or annually. You must include *everything*, no matter how insignificant it might seem.

You should not assume that costs are going to rise year on year. Fixed costs may not necessarily be 'fixed'. Look closely at each item in turn: is there any room for manoeuvre? Salaries probably make up a large proportion of your fixed costs. Are you able to reduce your wages bill?

Zero-based budgeting

I came across the concept of zero-based budgeting a number of years ago: I was an instant convert.

Traditional budgeting techniques are based on historical costs plus a percentage increase; this is known as incremental budgeting. The problem with this is that last year's figures are never questioned or analysed and therefore waste is perpetuated (sometimes ad infinitum). Dependence on past budgets assume that this year's objectives and strategies are the same as last year's. You should only use last year's budget as your first draft.

You could adopt a method of budgeting that starts with the assumption that *every* cost is unnecessary and that its inclusion in your budget therefore has to be justified. This is zero-based budgeting. Zero-based budgeting focuses on a close evaluation of each cost and on then prioritising them. The advantage of this technique is that you will be able to reduce or eliminate some costs altogether.

Hold this thought: zero-based budgeting makes you examine this year's objectives.

> Zero-based budgeting is so obvious. Instead of accepting that the cost of running the practice is inevitably going to rise year on year, I used to give myself the challenge of trying to bring it down. The result was I eliminated a great deal of waste and overspending on unnecessary materials. It also made me closely examine whether I was making best use of my employees. I bet that once you start drilling down into the running costs of your practice you find waste and overspending that you can eliminate.

If you prepared a budget last year, look at how it actually worked and at the variances. How much were your estimates out by, and why?

You must take into account the objectives you have set, together with any other factors that may have an impact upon the performance of the practice. What forecasts have you made about the demand for your services? How accurate do you think they are? If you are planning for growth, does your budget reflect this, or will you struggle to meet any extra demand?

No amount of planning and forecasting can accurately predict the future, but by taking time to consider every foreseeable eventuality you may just about get it right.

You should reflect on several questions.

- Has the practice set all of its objectives?
- Have you thought hard enough about the financial impact of each of them?
- Have you considered alternative (cheaper) strategies?
- Are there likely to be any changes from what you have planned?
- Are your income forecasts realistic or are they just wishful thinking?
- Have you included every possible item of expenditure?

What restraints are there likely to be?

Every practice has factors that limit its growth: it may be the physical size of the premises, their location or the lack of availability of suitable employees (dentists, hygienists, receptionists, and nurses). It could be that the competition for patients in your area is intense and therefore the number of potential patients is restricted.

A major restraining factor might be a lack of funds.

Growth is not always a good thing. It has to be financed, and even if in the long term it will (hopefully) produce increased profits, the effect on your cash flow has to be taken into account. You must ask yourself, 'If the practice does grow, how is that growth going to be accommodated, managed and financed?'

You need to ask yourself some financial questions.

- Where is the income going to come from to support the growth?
- Does it all have to be generated?
- Are you dipping into funds from a previous year?
- Is it borrowed money?

If you are relying solely on generated income, ask yourself:

- How accurate are your forecasts?
- How much of your income is guaranteed?

Don't rush headlong for growth unless you are absolutely certain that you have first considered the impact upon your short-term financial position and stability.

There is more on this in 'Planning to expand your practice' in Chapter 16 *Do more better*.

Financial control made easy

Your accountant is there to prepare your profit and loss accounts, your balance sheet and, if they are any good, to give you sound business advice. He or she will also be able to prepare a budget and cash-flow projection if you want them to. They will charge a fee. There is no reason, however, why you should not be able to prepare your budget and cash-flow projection yourself using the methods set out above. Doing so will certainly bring you closer to your business, and at the same time increase your understanding of how money 'works'.

Constantly review and work on your budget and cash-flow projections: rework your figures as you go along; revise your 'new' projections; work to keep within your budget through constant monitoring. Adopt a dynamic and, if needs be, an aggressive approach to managing your finances.

Hold this thought: it is cash flow and not profit that will ultimately determine whether your business survives.

> Having a budget, and reviewing it weekly, enabled me to see where I was spending my money. If costs needed to be reined in I was able to proactively do this rather than waiting until the cash had been spent, by which time it was too late.

Surviving the credit crunch and what followed

Before the world's financial institutions went into meltdown in 2008 credit was freely available. Almost overnight banks became very wary about lending to anyone. Former safe bets were now regarded as long shots, and that included dentists and their businesses.

Businesses that had been built on (excessive) borrowing and those with cash-flow problems suddenly became non-viable. As someone commented, an illusion of wealth had been built on a mountain of debt.

Which practices were best placed to beat the crunch and the recession(s) that followed? The survivors were those that:

- were very well managed *before* the credit crunch
- had low (or no) borrowings
- had a (very) positive cash flow
- had invested in a customer care programme (so held on to their customers)
- adjusted their product mix and prices in response to the rapidly changing economic environment (restaurants starting to offer two for one deals etc.).

Even in better economic times, having robust mechanisms in place by which your practice budget and cash flow are controlled makes sound management sense.

Finance, and having to think about money, is something a lot of dentists would prefer not to do, but unfortunately it is a necessary evil. However, you should not let money and profit become your sole driving force. Excellent customer service must always come first; money and profit will follow.

Hold this thought: in the early days of practice ownership you will owe more than you own. As time goes by you should own more than you owe, until eventually you owe nothing and own everything.

> I practised when interest rates were much higher than they are at present and at a time when they used to frequently fluctuate. I had business borrowings like most other practice owners, but whenever the interest rate on my loan fell, instead of letting my repayments also fall I used to *increase* my repayments; that way I repaid more of the capital quicker.

(*See* Chapter 11 *The practice manager.*)

15

Marketing planning

Developing your marketing plan

Much of the information you have gathered as part of the business planning process can be used to write a stand-alone marketing plan.

Before you embark on writing your plan there are some fundamental questions that need to be answered.

- What image do you think people in the town have of your practice?
- Can you change or improve your image?
- Have you definitely identified your competitors?
- What distinguishes you from your competitors?
- Can outside agencies help you with your marketing?

If you have tried 'marketing' before but had little or no success, was it because:

- it was unsystematic and haphazard
- you did not set measurable objectives or targets
- your objectives or tactics were not communicated to the rest of your team?

Having a marketing plan will help you avoid the pitfalls of approaching 'marketing' in a random fashion. Formalising your marketing plan will help you to:

- follow a rational path when making important decisions
- reduce potential conflicts and misunderstandings among the whole team
- leave the day-to-day implementation of your marketing strategies to your employees.

Compiling your marketing plan should not take long if you have already followed the steps outlined in the business planning process. It follows a similar pattern.

- Set (review) your practice objectives. Marketing is a function of your business objectives and not something separate.
- Carry out a marketing audit. Analyse and understand the environment in which the practice operates by carrying out a SWOT analysis. The strengths and weaknesses identify factors internal to the practice, while opportunities and threats identify external factors that the practice may have little or no control over but which, nevertheless, it must anticipate and evaluate.
- Make assumptions based on the past performance of the practice.
- Set your marketing objectives: define which treatments/products/services are to be sold in which markets.
- Estimate the expected results. These must be measurable and not simply statements about 'increasing' the number of patients, etc. Specify numbers for what you hope to achieve, e.g. 30 new patients per month.
- Formulate your marketing strategies. These describe the methods by which the marketing objectives are to be achieved, and they fall under four headings:
  1. product
  2. price
  3. place

4. promotion.

- Come up with an action plan for how each of your strategies is to be carried out.
- Everyone in the practice must both be told of the plan and understand it – don't just hand out written copies. Make a verbal presentation to your employees so you can inject *your* enthusiasm for the plan into *them*. If you do not communicate the plan to them and do not motivate them, there is the risk that the plan will fail.

When budgets are tight you need to look at using guerrilla tactics to help you achieve your marketing objectives. These are methods or new ways of thinking about how you can keep your practice in the public eye. Consider using the following approach.

- Don't spend your entire marketing budget on one campaign. Spread it over a number of smaller campaigns. People are more likely to remember you if they have seen your name in a number of different places and contexts. Use a 'drip, drip, drip' method.
- Go for frequency over size with your campaigns. Low-level marketing at regular intervals is more effective than a one-off massive campaign.
- Encourage your patients to spread the word about how good your practice is. Word of mouth marketing (such an apposite term for dental marketing!) is a powerful and absolutely free method of connecting with a great many potential new patients.
- Get the practice in the news (in a positive way). Local newspapers are often looking for local success stories to fill their pages. Help them out by telling them about your practice.
- Don't ignore your existing patients. It is pointless running a marketing campaign to attract new patients if you are losing the old ones because you are ignoring them.

If you have any patients who are journalists suggest ideas for stories related to your practice to them. Anything positive about you and/or your practice and your employees makes good copy.

> Editors of magazines, journals and publications of all shapes and sizes are constantly on the lookout for 'good copy'. I am often asked to write articles, and sometimes to come up with the idea for the article myself. If you want to get a story about your practice in to print, you should look for a new angle, something that captures the reader's attention and interest from the very beginning, and which leaves them wanting to know more.

Public relation consultants don't come cheap but, again, if one of your patients works in this field you might be able to glean some ideas from them or even obtain special rates if you engage them on a project-by-project basis.

Marketing is generally something that the majority of dentists either have no interest in or knowledge of, and therefore coming up with a marketing plan is likely to be seen as either time-consuming or unnecessary. If you really don't have any enthusiasm for marketing you could always bring someone in to help you and your practice manager if they too lack enthusiasm or the basic skills. I am not talking about hiring a consultant who will want to charge a hefty fee, but someone with the basic knowledge of what marketing is and how it works, and who has the time to write your marketing plan.

Most universities have a department of business studies and their final-year students generally have to carry out a case study, which does not have to be of a large business. Why not contact your nearest university and see if you can get one of their students to use your practice as their project? Even if there are no students available for this, there might be someone, possibly a postgraduate, who might jump at the chance to earn some extra money (student pay is a lot less than a consultant's!) while supplementing their studies. They could either work alongside your practice manager or work independently. They do not need to have access to patient records, so patient confidentiality is not an issue, but you would need to draw up a 'letter of engagement' that includes a confidentiality clause to protect your business ideas and your financial information.

Stick to the same rigorous recruitment process that you follow when looking for other employees. If you have not done so already, your marketing person could:

- devise questionnaires and carry out market research
- uncover the practice's strengths and weaknesses; outsiders often see what insiders prefer to close their eyes to
- research the competition and explore opportunities and threats
- write your marketing plan
- help come up with some cost-effective marketing strategies.

If it is a while since you put together your business plan or marketing plan, they could review them for you and maybe come up with some fresh ideas.

If you have recently put together these plans you might just want them to confirm that what you propose is feasible or whether there are any alternatives that you have perhaps overlooked. Fresh thinking is always a good thing.

> I got involved with the local university business school, which at that time was very actively promoting itself to local businesses.
>
> I had taken the practice through the whole business planning (and marketing planning) process, but I wanted some outside input into the finished product. One of the business school's Masters students used my practice as her case study. Using my plan as a starting point, she began by interviewing a random sample of the patients. She explored the strengths and weaknesses of the practice, and identified the opportunities and threats. She slightly modified my plans. It was a very worthwhile exercise for both parties: she got her Masters and I got confirmation that my plans were workable.

A failure to plan is often why marketing fails. This takes me back to the Japanese view of British management, the 'Ready, fire, aim' syndrome. You should always have done your research and your homework before you embark on trying to get the message out there.

What's the cheapest way of marketing your practice? The answer is simple: use your existing, and hopefully very satisfied, patients who, with a little bit of encouragement from you, can be made to sing your praises from the rooftops. Word-of-mouth marketing is the name of the game, but it does depend on your practice being able to deliver first-class customer service.

Here's a little maths question for you: if you had a tank that holds 1000 m³ of water, and you can fill it at the rate of 50 m³ per minute, how long will it take you to fill the tank? That's easy! 20 minutes. But what if the tank has a hole in it and is losing water at the rate of 20 m³ per minute; how long is it going to take you now? The answer is 33.33 minutes. Not only will it take you longer to fill your tank, but you will also have wasted over 660 m³ of water in the process, which if you are on a water meter, is going to cost you money.

So what's all that got to do with marketing? Well, sadly, a significant number of dentists waste vast sums of money every year (I've heard figures of £30k per annum being bandied around!) trying to entice more and more people into their practices through the front door, while ignoring the steady stream of patients who are walking out through the back door. When answering the maths question above, instead of working out rates etc., I would have said, 'Let's plug the hole!'

Dentistry is a very personal service, so why not make your marketing personal? When I was in practice I had nice patients and I wanted lots more nice patients just like them. There's always going to be 'leakage', so every practice needs if not a torrent, then at least a trickle of new patients, and if your existing patients are the type you want then why not encourage them to recommend their nice friends, nice family and nice work colleagues to you?

I had plastic, gold-coloured credit card-sized business cards made up (people tend not to throw plastic cards away, and they like gold), with my name and the practice's contact details on, which I handed out, three at a time, to my favourite patients at the end of their treatment session. I told them that one of the cards was for them to keep and the other two were for them to pass on to any friends, family and work colleagues who they thought might like to also benefit from being a patient of the practice. The personal touch was vital because it was an invitation from *their* dentist to recommend. I wanted to retain an air of exclusivity about the practice, so I added, 'Although the practice isn't actively looking for new patients, we would accept *your* recommendations.' This was a very personal invitation; I was taking my time (2 minutes at the end of an appointment) and was not delegating the job to a third party. But it did not stop there. I added that if any of their friends, relatives or work colleagues were to contact the practice, they had to say that they had been recommended by so-and-so. My team had their part to play in all this, because, first, they had to be prepared for an increase in new patient enquiries, and, second, they had to make a note of the sources of all new patients, and to greet them with a warm and sincere welcome. Everyone in the practice knew exactly what they had to do. I obviously thanked everyone who had recommended the practice at their next appointment.

Advertisements, mail drops, leaflet drops or banners don't work because they are not guaranteed to always reach your target audience. Besides which, how many leaflets that drop through your door do you actually read? Carpet-bombing an area is not the way to attract the right type of patients to your practice. Precision marketing that relies on your very satisfied patients being encouraged by you to spread the word about your wonderful practice is a much more cost-effective strategy. But if your level of customer care is dire, looking for new patients, any patients, simply means that all you will be doing is putting more people off. Nothing travels faster than bad news.

Hold this thought: whatever you do, before you go looking for new patients, make sure your existing patients are 110% satisfied.

None of this is new, but it works. It is a strategy that relies heavily on the personal touch and on everyone at your practice being able to deliver excellent customer care to new, as well as to existing, patients. So much marketing revenue is wasted because too much time and effort is spent chasing new business, while existing business is ignored and neglected.

Hold this thought: growing your patient numbers depends on building rapport with existing patients and on making a good first impression with new ones.

(*See* 'The practice manager as marketing manager' in Chapter 11 *The practice manager.*)

> I have a friend who uses much the same method of acquiring new patients, except that they will only ever accept new patients who have been referred by existing patients. I think they also exercise a ruthless policy of offloading patients they don't want.

16

Do more better

Planning for quality: doing the right thing right every time

Nothing wastes money, time and effort more than *not* doing the right thing right first time.

Having got your employees to 'buy in' to your practice philosophy, you might be tempted then to leave them to 'do their own thing'. This can be a dangerous strategy, but paradoxically showing them that you trust them to do their jobs right is a big step towards gaining their commitment to your practice and to ultimately running an effective and efficient operation. You must trust everyone to do the right thing right. However, there are a number of riders that need to be attached to this statement.

- Make sure that each employee knows that they are personally responsible for their own work.
- Remind them that they are part of a team and as such the standard of their work is going to be monitored by other employees (internal customers).
- The ultimate judge of their work, and of all the work carried out by the practice, will be the patients (external customers).
- You cannot possibly expect them to know what to do and how to do it unless they have been shown and told; better still, write it down!

> One practice manager said that she uses show and tell a lot when introducing new procedures, techniques, indeed anything new, into the practice. She realises that not all of the staff grasped the concept straightaway, so she does show and tell not once, not twice, but three times. She finds this tends to work.

This basic concept of doing the right thing right first time is the idea behind something called Total Quality Management (TQM), which you should incorporate into your practice as a systematic way of guaranteeing that everything that happens within the practice happens in the way it has been planned to happen.

In the context of your practice, TQM means that:

- the goal of the practice is to achieve total patient satisfaction
- patient requirements need to be established and responded to quickly and effectively
- all employees will concentrate on the *prevention* of problems in the workplace rather than a cure
- everyone is involved – all work done by employees and suppliers is part of a process that creates a product or service for a patient
- each employee is a customer for work done by other employees and has the right to expect good work from them and the obligation to contribute work of a high calibre in return
- the standard of quality expected within the practice is 'zero defects' or 'no failures' – everyone has to understand the standards required and the need to do it right first time
- sustained quality excellence requires continuous improvement
- continuous attention must be paid to educational, training and development needs
- high-quality performance will be recognised and rewarded
- quality improvement is best achieved by the joint efforts of all employees.

This again ties in employees, quality, patients and continuous improvement. There's no getting away from these if you want a successful practice.

Constantly telling new recruits about your practice policies and procedures should of course be part of their induction process. Constantly reminding *all* of your employees is also important; if you want everyone to remember them, they must be written down and, where appropriate, prominently displayed so that no one has any excuse for not being aware of them.

Your employees, whether they have worked for you for 5 days or 5 years, should know what they are supposed to do at the beginning, during and at the end of each working day, and how it is to be done.

(*See* Chapter 8 *Developing the core values of your practice.*)

Raising your game: developing the practice

The unexamined life is not worth living

(Ancient Greek aphorism)

What do we mean when we talk about 'developing a practice'? The *Oxford English Dictionary* defines 'develop' as *Become or make larger or more advanced.*

Unless you are going to let your practice remain as it is from the day you bought it to the day you sell it, you will at some point have to give some thought to how it can be developed.

There are several aspects to developing your practice.

- Developing yourself as a professional, a clinician, a businessman or woman but, most importantly, as a person. The person who steps out of dental school with letters after their name is far from being the finished article. You must be prepared to invest a great deal of time and effort (and money!) in self-development.
- Working with your employees, helping them and eventually the practice reach their full potential. Running a practice is a team effort.
- Developing the clinical services.
- Developing the business side of the practice.

All the above are intrinsically interlinked.

Developing yourself is perhaps the key to eventually having a successful practice. At one end of the spectrum there is going to be the superb clinician who is devoid of personality; at the other end there is the urbane, half-decent clinician; and then there is everything else in between. What patients want is a dentist they feel comfortable with, a confident (but not overconfident), competent, pleasant-to-talk-to, professional. Someone in whom they can put their trust.

You must develop your social and communication skills, and hence your ability to get on with people of all ages from different social and cultural backgrounds. Your ability to communicate well with various groups of people is critical.

Do you struggle to explain dental procedures and treatments to your patients? If this is you, practise talking about dentistry using everyday non-dental language. Do some types of patient render you tongue-tied? Why? Analyse who they are and what it is that makes you like this. Patients are now much more informed about dentistry, in fact about most things, because of the Internet. You must not feel challenged or in any way undermined when patients start to talk to you about things that you think they shouldn't know about. Go with it and let them help you give them the best advice and treatment appropriate for them.

As time goes by the clinical services you offer should improve technically and broaden. Even if you are a specialist, you still need to keep your knowledge of every other part of dentistry up to date. The qualitative and quantitative development of your clinical services is vital. Do you want to really go on offering more of the same?

Hold this thought: developing yourself as a manager and business owner is as important as developing your skills as a clinician.

> I enjoy learning new things, so when I was in practice I used to go on dental courses in which at first I had little interest, but which I told myself I should do to keep my clinical knowledge fresh and relevant. I threw myself into learning how to manage and how to be a better manager, and the skills I learned through this contributed a great deal to my personal development, and to my development as a writer and an expert witness. Nothing you learn is ever wasted.

Hold this thought: don't limit your intellectual stimulation solely to dental-related study.

Try to avoid becoming someone who does nothing but work and sleep, and, even worse, someone who only ever talks about their job. During the course of your working day you will have to make conversation with a number of different patients, all of whom lead varied lives and have varied interests and hobbies. Engaging in meaningful conversation with every one of them means you must have an interest in and know something about a very wide range of topics.

When it comes to developing your employees, at the very least you want them to possess qualities and qualifications relating to their ability to perform their role. However, you should want much more than that. You need to develop their customer care skills, their communication skills and their ability to get on with people of all ages from different social and cultural backgrounds. Helping a younger member of your team develop as a person, and watching them grow in confidence, knowledge and expertise, is very rewarding.

Continuous improvement of your employees, your practice, and of course yourself is the only way you are going to survive in the business of dentistry. One way in which this can be achieved, often quite rapidly, is through the process of benchmarking (comparing one thing with another that may be or may be not of a higher standard).

Many dentists work in isolation in the sense that they are not often exposed to the work patterns, methods or the techniques of their colleagues. It is therefore easy to quickly fall behind. Why not find a benchmarking partner and begin to regain some of the lost ground?

There are no real disadvantages to benchmarking, but there are four significant advantages:

- by choosing the right partner, performance goals are stretched
- it will accelerate any change programme
- it can motivate employees by showing them what is possible
- it is an early warning system of loss of competitive advantage.

> When I was thinking of specialising and of perhaps eventually having a specialist practice, I sought out a specialist practice (200 miles away from where I was, so no risk of competition) and spent several days there observing and absorbing. You should never be afraid of finding out that other practices are better than yours; that's how you learn and how to make yours better.

How do you begin the benchmarking process? There are several stages:

- identify exactly what it is you want to benchmark
- examine the process(es) you want to benchmark
- collect as much information about the process(es)
- identify your benchmarking partner(s)
- carry out the comparison exercise
- analyse the results
- formulate a plan to implement any improvements into your practice
- monitor and review.

Note how this process is the 'plan, organise, implement, review and monitor' cycle of management.

The things you may consider for benchmarking are 'hard' issues, such as clinical processes and procedures, and 'soft' issues such as management style, communications or customer focus.

Who you benchmark against can either be someone within your practice (if it is a large practice) or another practice. Practices in the same town may be unwilling to cooperate with someone they might

> I spent years fine tuning the standard of customer care in my business, and old habits die hard, I suppose. Now, even though I've long been out of business, I can't help tuning into how receptionists, waiters and waitresses, other professionals, and every retailer, speak to their customers. It costs nothing to treat customers properly and yet so many people still don't get it, do they?

see as a competitor. If yours is a general practice you could use a specialist practice (which does not see you as a competitor) as your benchmarking partner. You don't have to limit your benchmarking partners to similar practices; seeing how a highly regarded specialist practice operates, or even a non-dental organisation, can sometimes be very informative. Approach prospective partners and sell the idea to them on the basis that it will be a two-way process, so they will get something out of it as well. You must be willing to share information, but you will also have to consider the ethical issues involved, such as patient confidentiality and data security.

> When I was secretary of the Institute of Management Consultants we used to arrange visits to various businesses. I remember two in particular. The first was to the flagship store of a major supermarket: we went behind the scenes and, guided by one of their senior managers, got to see the lengths this business went to in order to make sure that their customers were the absolute focus of everything their staff did. The second was to an engineering company, something I'd never been inside before, but what an eye opener it was seeing the whole manufacturing process and the production of metal components to very exacting standards. Not unlike dentistry, really.

Planning for increased productivity

In the first edition I suggested that there were are a number of 'models' of the use of your time, your employees and the surgeries:

- one dentist, one nurse/receptionist and one surgery
- one dentist, one nurse, one receptionist and one surgery
- one dentist, two nurses, one receptionist and two surgeries
- one dentist, three nurses/receptionists and two surgeries.

Since I wrote that, CQC has rather changed all this, now that staffing levels have to be such that patient safety is not compromised, and also cross-infection control has to be far stricter than it ever was. Nevertheless, these models make a good starting point for you to begin to think about how you and your team could become more productive.

Hold this thought: as the dentist you are the one whose time is the most valuable, so it is important that you maximise its use.

Working with one nurse/receptionist and one surgery means that there are times when you will have to work on your own, which is not advisable for a number of reasons. In terms of your productivity, this is the worst scenario.

Having a nurse always on hand in the surgery, and a receptionist to answer the telephone and manage patients' appointments, means that you can get on with your work without your nurse having to continuously break off to deal with patients in reception. However, only having one surgery means that there are inevitable delays while you wait for the nurse to clear away and then prepare for the next patient. This, however, remains the model the majority of practices adopt.

If yours is a genuine private practice you may feel that once a patient is seated in your surgery you have to devote all of your time to them. Darting back and forth between patients, injecting one in one surgery and returning to another who is ready for you to begin work on may not appear to be good customer care. In a busy NHS practice this might be the only way you can get through the amount of work you have to do.

If you adopt the two-surgery model you have to have nurses who are able to 'fill the gap' if you are in the other surgery by talking to a patient. Patients must not be left alone in a surgery or they will feel abandoned. Well-trained and knowledgeable nurses can be invaluable salespeople, helping to reassure nervous patients, or educating them about the procedure they are just about to undergo. Patients are sometimes reluctant to ask the dentist about their treatment but will talk freely to a nurse.

Utilising two surgeries frees up time for emergencies and so enables you to offer an enhanced service.

> My practice went through several periods when it was in the doldrums. When I was younger and had a great deal of energy I used to make full use of the two surgeries I had and, for a short time, I worked very long days (8 a.m. to 7 p.m.). Hard work is sometimes the only way of keeping things going.

Organising your practice

When you moved into your practice you probably had to accept the layout of the reception, of the surgery(ies) and the relationship of one to the other. You may not have actually given any of this much thought. However, whatever physical restrictions there may be on the configuration, after a while you could give this some thought and think about how it could be modified to first improve productivity and, second, to improving the care of your patients.

You should never overlook the care of your existing patients, shuffling them backwards and forwards between reception, your surgery, the hygienist's surgery etc. The introduction (first impressions) of the new patient into the practice is equally important, and the way they are guided through the practice is something to which you should give some thought.

The through-flow of patients has to be seen in context of improving efficiency, but it also needs to be fitted around the efficient functioning of the clinical areas. The processes of setting up, clearing away, decontamination, rebagging etc. must all be taken into account when you are thinking about the planning and organisation of the practice.

> We used to discuss case studies (anonymised, of course) at our Institute of Management Consultancy meetings, and one case I remember well was that of how to improve the productivity of a production line that turned out such and such a component. The consultant involved told us how they had first observed how things were currently being done, carrying out a time and motion study as they went along. But rather than recommending one big change to the whole process, they had identified a number of stages where if small tweaks were made, the whole process could be made more productive and time-efficient. This was done and a significant percentage increase in output without any reduction in quality was achieved. This methodology could equally be applied to the process of treating and caring for patients, couldn't it?

Planning to expand your practice

Sic parvis magna (Greatness from small beginnings)

Sir Frances Drake's motto

What do we mean when we talk about 'expanding a practice'? The *Oxford English Dictionary* defines 'expand' as *Make or become larger or more extensive.* This may not mean that the physical size of the practice premises necessarily increases, or that more space within the practice is given over to the delivery of dental treatment. In what follows 'expansion' can mean one or all of an increase in patient numbers, and an increase in turnover and profit.

Before the *How?* of expanding a practice is tackled, you need to first revisit the *Why?*

To recap, your aims with any expansion programme should be to:

- increase your turnover
- increase your profit
- improve your cash flow.

Your budget and cash-flow projections for a period of planned growth (the emphasis is on planned) must always be very carefully thought through. I suggested in Chapter 14 that you can probably do these yourself, but if you don't feel you can, you are best getting your accountant to do it for you.

The potential financial problems that accompany any expansion are often insidious. The young, inexperienced or naïve practice owner can quickly find themselves in a precarious financial position.

But why can expansion be so harmful? Overexpansion relative to available resources (usually money) leads to a situation known as overtrading. Cash flow dries up and working capital has to be used to pay for materials, laboratory bills, wages etc. *before* the money from sales comes in. The speed at which this occurs depends on the rate of expansion and the amount of working capital you started off with. If you were running the business on an overdraft, this will rise, so increasing interest charges, perhaps also leading to new arrangement fee charges being incurred. If you didn't have an overdraft, you might soon have one! The business can quickly run out of money. Increasing interest charges affect your profit, which in turn reduces your working capital. A practice that was once financially stable can soon enter a cycle of financial instability and insecurity. Big is not always best!

I know of a long established and financially healthy business that for some reason thought it should expand by buying one of its competitors. It did this, but within 2 years it went out of business. A combination of bad management of the takeover, and probably a lack of cash afterwards, were the likely causes.

How can you avoid this?

- Plan any proposed expansion very carefully.
- Work through the financial impact with your accountant. This is not the time to go it alone.
- Don't overexpand!

Moving on to the *How?* of expanding a practice, there are two scenarios:

- organic growth of a single practice or of each practice within a group (hypertrophy)
- through the acquisition of other practices (hyperplasia).

There are four ways to expand a practice.

1. Find more patients.
2. Do more work on each patient.
3. Increase the value of your treatment(s).
4. Increase efficiency.

Not only do you want to find more patients, but also they must be the right type of patients. Stop and think: who or what is your 'ideal' patient? Is it someone who keeps his or her appointments, who turns up on time (usually a few minutes early!), never has any problems, doesn't talk too much so you are able to get straight on with their treatment, and who pays promptly? If you had a practice full of them you'd probably be happy. Applying the Pareto principle, probably 20% of your patients fit this description, so why not target them and encourage them to recommend their friends, relatives and work colleagues to you? Personal recommendation is a powerful marketing tool. Don't stop when you have replaced all of the problem patients with 'ideal' patients – you are, after all, expanding the practice!

Doing more work on each patient is another way of expanding your practice, but it raises ethical as well as business issues. What do we mean by 'more work'? A simple example (exaggerated, admittedly) could be someone who attends for a new patient examination: you have a look around his or her mouth, everything looks okay, so you say to them, 'I'll see you in 12 months.' You've earned the fee for a new patient examination, however much that is. Another scenario, with the same patient, could be: an examination that includes a periodontal assessment using a Basic Periodontal Examination probe (you find early pocketing around several molars), you take right and left bitewing radiographs (mesial caries, just into dentine, in one of the premolars) and upper and lower incisor periapical radiographs (no problems there), 'I see you've only got one tooth missing. Have you ever thought about having it replaced? I can talk to you about a bridge or possibly an implant if you want.' So now you'll be paid for a new patient examination, a referral to the hygienist to deal with the early periodontal disease, one restoration and possibly a bridge or an implant. None of this work is unnecessary, but it means you are doing more work on that patient and earning more money as a consequence. You might not be expanding your practice in terms of patient numbers, but you will be expanding it in terms of income and profit.

Increasing the price of your services is one way of expanding your turnover. The fee you charge for any item of treatment should reflect the cost of the materials (including any laboratory fees) and the time it takes, plus a 'profit'. Your accountant should be able to help you set or increase your fees.

The final way of expanding your practice is to increase the efficiency of what you do. You and your employees should always aim to get everything right first time.

Managing more than one practice

Expanding your business by increasing the number of practices you own is something you might think about doing. What are the potential benefits of owning more than one practice? There is possibly only one: increasing the turnover and hopefully the profits of the whole business. The problem is that you might create a second business that becomes difficult to manage or which becomes unmanageable because you are in effect having to manage it remotely, unless, of course, you employ a second practice manager, but even this can bring its own problems.

It is critical that before you consider buying or setting up a second practice you have excellent management systems and an excellent management team in place in your first practice that can be replicated in the second practice.

Hold this thought: don't take your eye off the ball and neglect your first practice.

You'd think it would be easy, replicating success and expanding your embryonic empire. I don't want to put you off the idea, after all people have done it, but the message I want to get across is that you should always learn to walk before you run.

Acquiring a second practice is as big a step as acquiring the first, except that you should by now have a better idea about how to manage a business. Buying or setting up a second practice follows the same process as when you bought or set up the first practice (*see* Chapter 3 *The process of buying an existing practice*), but let's look at what should happen before and after that, and let's think about it in terms of the management cycle of planning, organisation, implementation and control.

Under 'planning' you should:

- make the business case for having a second practice; talk it through with your accountant
- ask whether the two practices will work together as one entity or as two stand-alone sites
- work out where you are going to get your employees from, especially the clinicians
- decide whether you are going to work at the new practice, even if it is just on a part-time basis. You can't be in two places at once.

If the business case is not strong enough, don't proceed.

If the two practices are expected to function as one unit, how easily will it be to organise team meetings? If employees from your first practice are expected to work in the second practice, are you risking breaking up the team spirit you have spent so much time building?

Will your practice manager be expected to manage both sites? They also can't be in two places at once. If you decide to employ a second manager you will instantly be adding their salary to your wage bill.

These are just a few of the questions you should be asking, but once you have decided to go ahead, then the next stage is 'organising'.

Hold this thought: an excellent business plan is just as important second time around as it was the first time.

Organising is about gathering together all the resources needed to achieve the result. What resources are you going to need?

- People.
- Money.
- Strong management (I've included this because although it is not a tangible resource, it is nevertheless something you are going to need).
- A functioning dental practice and everything that includes.

People are often the biggest headache. First, you might have to put your trust in a new dentist; second, you might have to put your trust in a new nurse, a new receptionist, and a new practice manager, all of whom will be out of sight of you and your original practice manager.

Hold this thought: when the cat's away, the mice will play.

Provided you've taken your time to go through the planning and organisation stages, then implementation should not be too much of a problem. However, rather than leave the mice to play, I would give your original practice manager carte blanche to oversee and control what goes on in practice number two, at least in the early days.

There are practice owners who use one manager to manage across several sites. I have never thought this is a good thing; apart from anything else the manager is probably wasting valuable time travelling between the various practices. One manager per practice makes more sense, but then there is the cost implication as well as there being consistency in the quality of the management.

Managing disaster

Business Continuity Management (BCM) is something that needs your serious attention.

What would be the impact on your business if your premises burnt down or they suffered long-term flooding, or if one night an articulated lorry ploughed into the front of the building? Would you or your employees know what to do to ensure that your business was able to continue, let alone survive?

There are several steps to continuity planning.

- Analyse the risks to your business. Where is the business vulnerable? What would be the effect on the service(s) you provide:
  1. in the first 24 hours?
  2. in 24–48 hours?
  3. within 1 week?
  4. in 1 to 2 weeks?
  5. in the longer term?
- Assess the risks. For each risk you identify you then need to ask three simple questions.
  1. How likely is it to happen?
  2. What impact will it have on my practice and my business?
  3. What can I do to reduce the likelihood or effect or to mitigate the risk entirely?
- Develop your business continuity strategy. You could:
  1. do nothing
  2. accept the risks, but make arrangements with other practices for help
  3. reduce the risks, but still make arrangements as above
  4. reduce the risks to the point where you do not need help.
- Develop your plan, which should contain these key areas:
  1. roles and responsibilities
  2. incident checklists for key employees

3. what must be done in the first hour
4. things that can wait
5. how often your plan will be reviewed.

You will need to build into your plan additional information from outsiders such as:

- your landlord
- neighbouring practices and other businesses
- utility companies
- your insurance company
- suppliers
- the Local Authority Emergency Planning Officer
- emergency services.

Finally, you should test and rehearse your plan.

In the final analysis, your Business Continuity Plan (BCP) has to address two issues: people and premises.

Writing your BCP is relatively straightforward. It will need to contain the following information:

- a list of all of the people who have been given a copy of the plan
- an analysis of the impact in the first 24 hours, 24–48 hours, up to 1 week and beyond
- the resources needed for recovery in each of these timescales
- a list of priorities
- an emergency response checklist
- a list of key contacts and their contact details
- a log sheet to tick things off as they are done.

Don't keep all of the copies of the plan in the practice.

Planning for something that might never happen may seem like a pointless exercise, but if disaster does strike, being prepared for it means that the practice will recover much quicker than it otherwise would. You may think that your patients would 'bear with you' while you take ages to find somewhere suitable to treat them; the reality is that they may not want to wait that long.

Hold this thought: the most perfectly constructed system is occasionally subject to malfunction (Hans Fallada in *Alone in Berlin*).

Section V

Policies and procedures

This section could be as short as three words, 'WRITE EVERYTHING DOWN!', that is, after you've shown and told, but that would not help you to understand why everything must be written down. The importance of writing everything down is that, in the long term, it will make your life easier.

It is important that you understand the difference between 'policy', which is defined as 'a course of action adopted by an organisation or person', and 'procedure', which is defined as 'an established or official way of doing something' or 'a series of actions done in a certain way'. For example, your practice *policy* regarding the handling of patient complaints might state that all patient complaints will be resolved to the patient's satisfaction. Your patient complaints *procedure* sets out the stages involved in achieving this.

If you or any of your employees worked for a big, non-dental organisation, for example a bank or a large high street retail chain, everything you did during your normal working day would be set out in writing. How to open a current account or how to deal with a returned faulty item of clothing would all be meticulously documented. Company policy tells the employee what to do, and the procedure tells them how to do it. Successful organisations try not to leave any room for mistakes when it comes to their employees interacting with their customers. (Despite this, they still sometimes get it wrong because no one has bothered to train the staff.) Your practice should be no different in so far as everything must be written down; you should also train your staff.

For many years dental practices were unregulated, but now they are heavily regulated, so the need to have policies and procedures, and to comply, has never been more important.

17

Policies

What things do you need policies for?

It might be hard to believe, but at one time you did not have to have a policy for *any* aspect of your practice. Things are very different now. I have not even attempted to compile a list of the policies you must have, and the best advice is for you to keep up to date with any changes or additions as best you can.

Even in those areas where you are not legally required to have a policy, it is still good practice to have one because:

- employees will understand what is expected of them
- policies foster a culture of consistency.

It is always better to have a policy than to not have a policy.

Apart from having to have policies that relate to general business issues, there are also ones that are obligatory in dental practice, for example:

- cross-infection control
- radiation protection
- child protection
- handling patient complaints
- patient safety.

This list is nowhere near exhaustive and is likely to change over time, so, once again, always check that you are keeping up to date and legal.

You could, of course, buy all of your practice policies 'off the shelf', but if you do this there is a risk that you don't actually read them, and if you don't, are you really going to understand them? At dental school you bought textbooks and, yes, you will have read them, but to gain real understanding I bet you went through each one creating your own notes. This is all part of helping you learn and understand what you need to know. The same applies to policies; you have to understand what each one is about, and that is best done by writing them out yourself.

There are some general principles to which you should always adhere whenever you write a policy document.

- Always write them using simple, clear, and concise language.
- Avoid jargon and overly technical descriptions.
- Assume that the reader has no knowledge of the thing about which they are reading.
- Make it clear why the reader is going to need the information contained in the policy document.
- Date the policy.
- Update and review *all* policies on a regular basis.

Set your policies out as individual documents, but also incorporate them all into your practice manual. Employees must be made aware of them, especially during their induction process. Policy documents should be freely accessible by the employees and they must also be made aware of any changes as soon as they occur.

If you are going to introduce a policy into your practice there are several things you first need to consider.

- What is the purpose of the policy?
- Have you discussed its introduction with your employees?
- Who will have overall responsibility for the policy?
- Are there any costs associated with its introduction?
- How are you going to monitor and control the policy once it has been introduced?

Hold this thought: it is not sufficient to communicate change; the decision on which it is based must also be communicated.

How to write a policy document

If the thought of having to write a practice policy document fills you with trepidation, it might help if you think of it as consisting of four simple stages.

- Planning: you need to collect as much information as you can from as many sources as possible. Seek the opinion and view of your employees (they are more likely to accept the policies if they have been consulted). Talk to organisations closely linked with the subject of the policy.
- Development: write, and where necessary, modify the policy to suit the specific needs of your practice.
- Implementation: tell your employees that the policy has come into force. Provide additional training if necessary.
- Review: continuously monitor to make sure that the policy is being used correctly.

Always check that any policies you introduce, or modifications that are made, are not unlawful or discriminatory.

Even if you use off-the-shelf policies, it is critical that you and your employees spend time studying them to bring you all closer to what is going on right from the start.

18

Procedures

Why you need procedures documented

How your employees carry out their roles is more likely to be in accordance with your wishes if they have written guidelines to follow.

Delegating a team member to explain procedures to other employees does not always ensure that tasks will be carried out as they should be – people forget or misunderstand. Even if you, personally, take the time to explain things to them, people still forget. Having written procedures for your employees means that you do not have to be involved in the process of repeatedly telling them things, which is not a good use of your time; it is much more effective and efficient to have everything written down.

You could periodically include discussion of procedures as an agenda item in your team meetings.

Predictability and consistency in the outcome of everything that is done within the practice makes for a relatively stress-free life. Employees are more likely to deal with patients in the way you want, and not as the employee thinks they can or should be dealt with. Materials should be used as they are meant to be used, that is, according to the manufacturer's instructions; instruments and machinery are less likely to be broken through mishandling or inappropriate use.

How to write a procedure document

Writing a procedure document is not as difficult as you might think. Management is about getting things done through other people, so here is how you can get your employees to do it for you:

- produce a pro forma that asks the questions Who? What? Why? When? How? Where?
- give a number of these to each employee and ask them to fill one in for every task they do during a normal working day, e.g. the decontamination and sterilisation of instruments; registering a new patient
- when they have done that, get them to swap the pro forma with each other
- have each employee see if they can both follow the instructions and perform the tasks as set out on each pro forma
- modify as needed until each 'instruction' is crystal clear.

Try to standardise the layout of the sheets.

The aim is for someone who is not familiar with or who has no knowledge of a particular task to be able to complete it correctly simply by following what has been written down.

Hold this thought: how many products, even for the home, have instructions with them? Producers wrongly assume that people already know how to use their product(s).

When you (and/or your practice manager) are happy with the pro formas, type them up into finished copies. Don't forget to date them.

It should take you no more than a couple of weeks to produce a written procedure for every task that every employee does during their normal working day. It is important that procedures are written down in very clear language, with no ambiguities or room for misinterpretation.

Each procedure document should be located in the part of the practice where that particular procedure takes place. However, you should also pull all your procedures together and incorporate them into your practice manual.

You and your practice manager should periodically review every policy and procedure to check whether or not it still complies with your current practice. If you change anything you must make sure that everyone in the practice knows and that they familiarise themselves with the new version.

When all of your policies and procedures have been written down you are ready to build a reference file, perhaps as described below.

- Use an A4 ring binder or lever arch file.
- Print a cover and spine label that reads 'Practice Policies and Procedures'.
- Number each page of each policy and procedure as 'X of Y'.
- Produce a sheet that lists the policies and procedures included in the file. This goes at the front of the file.
- Date each page as 'Last modified DD/MM/YYYY'.
- You should have two manuals in the practice manager's office, one that is the definitive (master) copy and one copy to lend to new recruits during their induction period – one copy in reception, and one in each of the surgeries.

Whenever a policy or procedure is altered or amended, the practice manager should be responsible for researching and recording the new one, including the date when it was last modified, and for removing and replacing old copies with new ones in *all* of the files. This is important because if this is not done your files soon become out of date, obsolete and meaningless.

How to write a practice manual

Your practice manual is a compendium, a reference book for everyone that works at the practice. It must therefore always be relevant and current. Because the manual is a reference document you should have paper copies available within the practice.

The great thing about having a practice manual is that it keeps all of your practice information in one place, which is accessible to everyone in your team.

What should you include and how should it be set out? The first thing to remember is that the manual should only contain those things that are already known within the practice:

- policies
- procedures
- standards of employee behaviour and conduct
- how performance is assessed.

Break the manual into sections.

- Introduction: this should tell the reader
  - what they are about to read
  - why they should read it.
- Section 1: General information about the practice – you might want to include the practice's mission statement, its core values and its charter. You want the reader to be impressed by how much the practice is dedicated to serving its patients. In a large practice it is a good idea to include the organisational structure of the practice, which is particularly useful and important for new recruits.
- Section 2: The practice manager – include a copy of the job description and a summary of the role and its responsibilities.
- Section 3: The receptionist – include a copy of the job description and a summary of the role and its responsibilities.
- Section 4: The dental nurse – include a copy of the job description and a summary of the role and its responsibilities.

- Section 5: The hygienist/therapist – include a copy of the job description and a summary of the role and its responsibilities.

Expand this basic list to include other roles if necessary.

Remember to update the manual as things change.

Have two copies in the practice manger's office: one as the practice master copy and one to give to new recruits as part of their induction. Give one to each employee (make sure they return it if they leave!). Have them sign to say that they have read it and keep this note in their employee file. There can then be no excuses for any of them not knowing about anything related to their job and to what goes on in the practice.

It might take you a while to initially assemble your policy and procedure, and practice manual, but once you have them they are invaluable tools that will help you manage your practice on a day-to-day basis without you having to be always personally involved. Great for time management and a must for reducing your stress levels!

In this highly technological age, there are companies who will provide you with just about everything you need to manage your practice online. This would seem to take a great deal of the stress out of the whole business. My concern is that by devolving such an important part of your business to a third party you risk losing a certain amount of involvement, which may not always be a good thing.

19

Compliance

Before the advent of CQC there were several routes down which practices could go to achieve accreditation, which basically gave them proof of competency and credibility. The accreditation bodies are still around, and it is worthwhile examining exactly what accreditation from each of them would mean to your practice.

Investing in your employees' development and training pays huge dividends in terms of helping your practice achieve its business objectives. This is the goal of Investors in People (IiP).

Gaining the IiP award will:

- publicly demonstrate the practice's commitment to training and development
- help you recruit and retain the right calibre of employee
- give you the framework for developing and improving the practice's skill base.

There are several principal requirements that the practice must satisfy before it will be awarded the IiP standard.

- It must make a public commitment to develop its employees. This commitment should be written into the practice's strategic plan. The commitment also requires everyone in the practice to know the broad aims of the business, understand the mission statement, and understand that the practice is committed to their development.
- There are regular reviews of the training and development needs of every employee. These needs are to be regularly reviewed against the practice's business objectives.
- There is continuing action to train and develop employees on recruitment and throughout their employment. This means the practice must have an induction programme.
- The investment made in training and development is regularly evaluated to assess its value in terms of the contribution to helping meet business objectives.

I hope this all sounds very familiar.

IiP can be a very useful management tool in terms of the training and development of your employees, but it comes at a price.

- Time. It can take a great deal of time to gain IiP, anything up to 1 year and sometimes up to 2 years.
- Energy. Not gas or electrical, but people's energy.
- Money. The assessment will cost money, as will any ongoing support and staff training.

There is nothing preventing your practice embracing the principles of IiP and making a commitment to develop and train its employees without having to submit to formal IiP assessor scrutiny. Why not discover if you have any patients who have at some time been involved with IiP? Perhaps they'd be prepared to help you. Training, developing and supporting your employees is a requirement of CQC, so maybe you could find someone who used to work for IiP to help you with CQC.

The International Organization for Standardization (ISO) is the family of quality systems that most people in business either work with or are at least aware of.

Whole books have been written about ISO, but in essence it is a set of requirements that include:

- procedures that cover all key processes in the business
- monitoring to ensure that they are effective
- maintenance of adequate records
- quality control with appropriate corrective action where necessary

- regularly reviewing individual processes and the quality system itself for effectiveness
- continuous improvement.

If you decide to seek ISO accreditation the practice would have to be independently audited. This costs money. There is also an ongoing annual fee for re-certification. What you should bear in mind, however, is that certification to an ISO standard does not guarantee the quality of end products or service; it merely certifies that formalised business processes are being applied.

IiP and ISO are not business specific in so far as they are meant to be for every type of business in every type of industry. However, gaining accreditation under one of these banners signifies to the wider business community that you run an excellent business and not just an excellent practice.

The British Dental Association (BDA) has its own quality assurance programme specifically for all dental practices, NHS, private, specialist and general, called The BDA Good Practice Scheme, or Good Practice for short. Like ISO, membership of the scheme does not guarantee the ongoing delivery of quality dental care; it is about the management of the practice.

There are probably four key benefits to being a Good Practice practice.

- It helps the practice perform to recognised standards of good practice.
- It promotes quality assurance.
- It helps build a motivated team.
- It is an excellent marketing tool.

At the heart of the scheme is a commitment to excellent practice management and to excellent patient care.

Naturally there is a cost involved in becoming a Good Practice practice.

You must explore each of these accreditation schemes yourself, and only when you are totally satisfied that the one you choose is going to bring you a significant competitive advantage over other practices should you commit.

If you do become accredited you must wring as much benefit (from a marketing point of view) as you can from it. All three schemes come with a plaque that you can hang in your reception area; they all allow you to incorporate the relevant logo onto your headed notepaper and practice literature. However, all of this might be a lost opportunity unless you tell your patients how and why the practice being accredited is going to directly or indirectly benefit them. Talk to them about your commitment to the training and development of your employees, and how the practice is ensuring patient safety by satisfying the standards set by, for example, CQC, the GDC, the Department of Health, and the Health and Safety Executive. I've suggested you tell your patients what a great employer you are and how you invest time, effort and money in training and developing your employees.

There is a saying among fiction writers that a writer should 'Show, not tell', so better than telling your patients, *show* them what a great employer you are by having a superb team around you. This may seem to contradict the practice of marketing, which is all about telling people about the benefits; however, 'showing' quite simply reinforces this message. The two go hand in hand.

Every practice now has to be a 'CQC' practice, or the equivalent in other parts of the UK, but if you do achieve Good Practice or any other of the general business accreditation, share this news with

---

I considered ISO but felt that it was not relevant to my practice.

We went a long way down the path towards IiP accreditation, but in the end my employees and I decided that we didn't need it.

In the end we opted for the BDA's Good Practice. I put the shiny plaque up in reception and told every one of my patients what being a Good Practice would mean for them. I think it reassured my existing patients but it did not bring new patients flocking to the door.

I'm not sure I would go down the accreditation route again. Having to comply with CQC is probably enough for most practices to cope with without having to satisfy other schemes.

I saw an advert for a private medical practice that claimed that they were somehow different, better than your run-of-the-mill NHS GP practice, by mentioning that their practice was registered with the CQC. Not quite misleading, but if all practices have to be registered it doesn't really make them better, does it?

the wider public. If you have a local newspaper, write a short piece for it setting out what the practice has achieved, briefly how it went about it, and what it will mean for patient care in the future. It is the benefits people are interested in, nothing else. (If you feel you would be unable to write such a piece, find someone who can.) This is all good marketing and, what is more, it is free! Most newspapers and local magazines are always looking to fill up their column inches, and if you can help them do this, so much the better.

Governance, or as it is now more commonly called, compliance, has been part of dentistry in particular and medicine in general since as long ago as the early 1990s, but historically it has its roots in the world of commerce.

What is compliance? Compliance means that you conform to a rule, a standard, a policy or a law. Most definitions include the improvement of, or at least the maintenance of, services, care and clinical standards. Is it not simply about doing the right thing?

Mentioning compliance often elicits reactions ranging from boredom or frustration, right through to cynicism and in some instances downright hostility from most dentists. However, whatever your view of it, it is probably here to stay. Learning how to work with it and understand how it could improve your practice is probably the easier option, rather than fighting against it.

Under the compliance umbrella sits auditing, which is the main method by which quality is monitored. So auditing something is simply checking to see that what is supposed to happen has actually happened; auditing what is supposed to happen in your practice is the only way you can maintain an overall high standard of management (in its broadest sense). There are two types of auditing:

- external – usually carried out by an external accreditation body
- internal – carried out by internal employees who have been trained to carry out this process.

The purpose of any audit is to continually review and assess, to verify that the system is working as it is supposed to, to find out where it can be improved, and to correct or prevent any problems that are uncovered.

When someone carries out an audit they want to know three things.

- Tell me what you do, i.e. describe the process.
- Show me where it says that, i.e. show me where it says that in the procedure manual.
- Prove that that is what happened, i.e. show me the evidence in documented records.

In the same way as you put together your policy and procedure manual, and your practice manual, so you need to put together an audit manual. The manual should consist of four sections, namely:

- policy
- processes
- references
- checks.

Checks should be carried out periodically to see that policies are being implemented and that processes are being followed. For example, you could check 10 randomly selected records of patients

---

i used an external auditor, someone who had been involved with IiP and so was familiar with the concept of auditing, to carry out 3-monthly audits of my patient records. It took a couple of hours and did not cost very much.

She always wrote me a short report listing her findings and recommendations, for example:

2.7 Record keeping – reference 5.4

From the sample taken, two patient records did not have information relating to tobacco and/ or alcohol use recorded (patient records xxxx and xxxx).

Action: there is currently a backlog of patient information waiting to be input, which may account for these omissions. I recommend that the backlog be cleared as a matter of urgency and a system for regular input maintained.

The problems she uncovered enabled me to improve my record keeping and to improve my patient care.

seen in the last 3 months, and whether they were new or old patients and note if a medical history had been taken.

You could, of course, simply buy an off-the-shelf compliance pack from a provider that tells you they can do everything for you. My concern about this is that by devolving such an important part of your business to a third party you risk losing a certain amount of involvement, which may not always be a good thing. Knowing about and keeping up with compliance issues is the responsibility of the practice owner. You won't do this if you aren't that close to it.

20

Managing the Care Quality Commission

I have resisted the temptation to cite CQC regulations, standards or whatever they might happen to be called, and have instead tried to set out a general-principle framework for you to work with and adapt to suit the circumstances at the time.

Before you read any of this chapter, you must first have read and absorbed the CQC's current guidelines, either in hard copy or on their website (their website is likely to be more up to date). You should be able to quote CQC in your sleep.

You must know the background to what is coming up in this chapter.

Hold this thought: with something like CQC, it is better to know too much than too little.

What is the CQC and what does it do? CQC is the regulator for all health and social care in England. In Scotland, this role is performed by Scotland's National Care Standards. In Wales, this role is performed by the Care and Social Services Inspectorate Wales. The equivalent body in Northern Ireland is the Regulation and Quality Improvement Authority. No matter in which part of the UK you work, there is a regulator overseeing what you do and how well you are doing it.

For convenience, I will only make reference to CQC, but the principles underpinning the work of the other regulators will, I am sure, not be dissimilar.

For a new practice, registering with CQC is the first thing you must do, and you should liaise with CQC to see how you should go about this.

Implementing and complying with CQC is probably the biggest piece of managerial work your practice will ever have to undertake, and whether you are implementing CQC for the first time in your new practice, or whether you want to ensure that you do not fail an inspection, you should first tackle this by following the four simple stages or steps of any management process.

1. **Planning:** first, you decide on a particular course of action to achieve a desired result. What is it you want to achieve? Initially, it is to register with CQC, then you want to comply and, finally, you want an outstanding rating at each and every inspection.
2. **Organising:** next, you gather together all of the resources you will need to achieve the result(s). What resources are you going to need? You are going to need paper, people and proof.
    *   Look on the CQC website and see what they say you must have and do to comply.
    *   Consult with any organisations of which you are a member who provide information and guidance about CQC compliance. (However, I would still use CQC material as your primary source.)
    *   Review your employee training plans – have they all completed appropriate training and, if so, where's the evidence? If you are a new practice, do the plans reflect CQC requirements for future compliance?
    *   Do all of your employees know what CQC is and their role in helping you comply? If not, it is now time to make sure they do.
3. **Implementing:** you then get other people to work together smoothly and to the best of their ability as part of a team to do the work.
    *   Break CQC up into manageable chunks then delegate pieces of work to individuals.
    *   Set a timescale for the delivery of each item.
    *   Then, finally, and working together, the whole team sets about reviewing and revising the material before it can present the final versions as evidence of compliance.

- You might decide that you'd like to perform a dry run, a dummy inspection, in which case draft in someone with the necessary knowledge and skills to act as the inspector.
4. Controlling: finally, you monitor, review or measure the progress of the work in relation to the plan and take steps to correct things if they are off course.

Hold this thought: once your team understands CQC, it will be much easier for your practice to comply.

If you follow this logical approach, completing the application form and registering with CQC should not pose too many problems. What takes the time, however, is the preparation of the evidence you are going to need to demonstrate that you are compliant with all of the regulations. The aim of each of these regulations is so that everyone using healthcare services has a positive experience that can be measured against a single regulatory framework, which, even without CQC watching over you, should be your aim in any event.

All of the CQC regulations appear to be common sense if what you hope to run is an exceptional practice. Although if everyone is achieving these standards, you are going to have to work extra hard making your practice stand out from the crowd.

Here are some easy ways in which you can start compiling the evidence and demonstrating compliance.

Before I move on, I think it is important to think of the way you manage CQC as being a two-pronged strategy. The first is to manage the process in house: the second is to bring in expertise (and use other people's time) if the whole process becomes too onerous.

If you have a practice manager, work out a plan together. Once you've done this, bring in all of the staff and get everyone involved with registration. As with everything else in your practice, managing CQC and getting it to work for you, is about teamwork, so the first thing to do is to make employees aware of CQC, breaking it down into manageable chunks so as not to overwhelm them. Understanding and knowing how CQC works is very much about your employees developing their management skills. I hope that by now you see that it is important that everyone in the practice acquires the skills of planning, organising, implementing, and reviewing, monitoring or controlling and that everyone understands how their workplace functions. Besides which, when the inspector calls they will want to talk to your staff: your staff will be better able to answer their questions if they have been involved in the processes right from the start.

Hold this thought: everyone working for you has to be a manager.

Start off with the CQC regulations and divide up the collecting of information among the relevant members of staff. Start off with a robust policy for each of the regulations, all supported by a comprehensive policy and procedure document, which all demonstrate compliance. The type of evidence you should be looking for could be in results from any relevant audits, surveys you'd carried out, logs of any activity, and contracts with outside agencies or contractors.

Hold this thought: your evidence must all be current evidence, and it is up to you to prove you are compliant.

To test if the evidence you hold is robust enough to demonstrate compliance, ask yourself.

- Is it current? (Within 12 months or longer if a long-term focus?)
- Is it reliable? (Is the source credible, is the evidence consistent, can it be validated or triangulated with another source?)
- Is it relevant? (Is it related to the regulations, the regulated activities and CQC's remit?)
- Is it sufficient? (Is there an adequate amount of evidence with enough detail to make an assessment?)
- Does it demonstrate the quality of outcomes and experiences of people using your services?
- Does it demonstrate what controls (processes) you have in place?
- Is specialist input (e.g. pharmacy, medical etc.) required?

What do you now need to do to ensure that your practice remains compliant?

Develop an annual action plan for policy reviews, staff appraisals, clinical audit, patient surveys, and building repairs to ensure safety and suitability of the premises. Have this plan available for the CQC inspectors when they visit. Why? Because when the inspector calls, and says they have concerns about, for example, an absence of clinical audit, then as long as your action plan shows that clinical audit has already been highlighted and that clinical audits are planned with a confirmed timescale for completion, you'll be fine. The fact that you have identified and planned for remedial action to rectify the situation is sufficient.

Hold this thought: if you haven't written it down it hasn't happened!

Assuming that you've got on top of CQC and you have everything in place, and all the necessary paperwork is filed nicely away in your office, the next thing to think about is the practice inspection. Inspections fall into three categories:

1. Scheduled
2. Responsive
3. Themed.

A scheduled inspection is part of the CQC's rolling programme of inspection.

A responsive inspection is when concerns have been raised about aspects of your practice.

A themed inspection is one where the inspector looks at specific areas, e.g. child protection.

It does not matter what type of inspection it is, or even the name CQC gives to it, you must make sure you are ready. The best time to start preparing for the next inspection is the minute after the inspector has finished the current one.

In the days when you had to trail off to the post office to tax your car, you had to take along your vehicle registration documents, your insurance certificate, and an MOT certificate if your car was more than 3 years old. I used to hate this because no matter how careful I'd been about filing away all of the above, when the day came you could bet that there was always one important piece of paper missing. Panic ensued while I frantically hunted everywhere. I became so paranoid that I used to check periodically that I could lay my hands on the documents even when I didn't need to. This is what a CQC inspection could be like if you don't file every bit of paper away in its proper place and if you don't know where that proper place is. If it were me I would, say, every couple of months, want to see all of the relevant CQC paperwork.

CQC inspection day should be like any other working day, so still see patients. Part of a CQC inspection is talking to patients, who could be asked about any aspect of the care and service they receive from you and your team. You cannot control what patients say, but if you and your team are all doing your jobs well they should not say anything negative, should they? At least you might get a chance to discuss the patient's comment with the inspector, which demonstrates your willingness to listen and consider ways in which your service could be improved. Hopefully, your practice is so brilliant that no one can ever come up with anything negative to say. If the inspector is obviously not fully conversant with how a dental practice operates and they come out with remarks and comments that seem unreasonable or irrelevant, rather than getting embroiled in a major row, try to have a rational discussion, while gently pointing out what should be really happening.

Following the inspection, which might only last a couple of hours, the inspector has to go away and write a report, which is then sent to you.

Your practice will be rated according to CQC's current regulations, and will be graded as follows.

- Outstanding (a green star) if it is performing exceptionally well.
- Good (a green traffic light) if it is performing well and meeting CQC's expectations.
- Requires improvement (an amber traffic light) if it isn't performing as well as it should be and CQC have told the practice how it must improve.
- Inadequate (a red traffic light) if it is performing badly and CQC have taken action against the provider.

- Unrated (a grey spot) for practices that can't for various reasons be rated.

All CQC reports are published on the Internet and so are in the public domain, to be read by everyone and anyone, including your current patients and some potential patients. It makes good business sense to always aim for a green star.

The inspector will talk to your employees, which might fill you with dread, wondering if they are going to say the right thing, but not if you have rehearsed their lines with them beforehand. The inspectors want to know about staff training: '*Have you had training in such and such?*' If they have, that's fine, but if they haven't they should not say they have.

The inspector will basically want to know if staff training has taken place to support each of the CQC standards. As part of your practice meetings and training sessions work your way through each of the standards and check to see if training has been carried out for each one. If it hasn't, do something about it. You can be sure that if you leave something out that will be the one thing the inspector will ask about. Staff training and development should not only be about the business objectives, you should train and develop with one eye on those all-important CQC standards. What good is CQC apart from having to do it?

You want your existing patients to know that they are in safe hands. You want potential patients to single out your practice as being better than the others. For example, you need to update staff resuscitation training, so why not contact the local newspaper, get them to send one of their photographers to the training session? Use the training session as a photo opportunity to promote your practice in the local newspaper and on your practice website to show how well trained your staff are. If you use a photograph taken by a professional photographer, you must ask their permission, and they will usually want some words of acknowledgment to go alongside the photo.

When you've carried out your annual patient survey, and you've found that 9 out of 10 patients would recommend the practice, isn't this something you should share with potential patients?

Hold this thought: don't be shy about telling potential patients how happy your existing patients are with your practice.

Mention of 'CQC' does sometimes strike fear into the hearts of practice owners and practice managers. The best advice, as with anything, is, first, don't panic; next, read all of the guidance material you can lay your hands on; share the process with your employees. Finally, you probably comply with most of the regulations already; you just have to have current, applicable evidence and robust policies to prove it.

I identified the same critical elements that CQC uses (I called them: employees, quality, patients, and continuous improvement, plus that all important one, communication) long before CQC came along. You too should look for new ways in which you can make your practice stand out from the rest.

21

Managing change

So you've read this book and you have decided you are tired of your practice as it is and that you feel that you need to make radical changes. Before you take a leap in the dark, however, a cautionary word: business planning does bring about change, but if you do not manage the change process well then it will fail and you could end up being worse off than if you'd left things the way they were.

The *Oxford English Dictionary* defines change as 'Make or become different'. That is what you have decided to do, to make your practice different from what it is now.

Where do you start? You must first recognise that all change affects people and that people generally don't like change, and some positively hate it. Change challenges their values.

You then have to accept that you cannot force change on your employees. If they are not convinced of the need for change or if they do not agree with how it is being carried out, there is real risk that they will leave. So before you embark on a big change, think back to when you tried to introduce a small change; who didn't like it?

You should begin your change programme by first mapping it out in general terms as outlined below; each stage of which must be fully thought through.

- Begin by recognising the practice's current set of values and culture.
- Outline what you hope the practice will look like at the end of the change programme. Set out your vision of the future.
- Make a case for change. *You* might know why the practice has to (must) change, but you have to convince others, to make it happen.
- Define the things that are going to change and the order in which you want them to change. Draft out a rough time-plan.
- Consider how the proposed changes are going to affect each employee, both personally and professionally. Are you going to have to invest more in training to help your employees cope with more demanding roles?
- Examine the financial cost.
- Draw up a list of the things that could inhibit the change.
- Don't forget to involve your employees.

Depending on the extent and nature of the proposed change you might either oversee its implementation yourself, delegate it to your practice manager, or both assume responsibility. It is nearly always preferable that you and your practice manager work alongside each other. This usually helps to overcome or at least minimise any resistance that is likely to arise from the other employees. Of course, if your practice manager expresses doubts, these must be addressed and dealt with *before* the proposed change is presented to others.

Implementing your change programme, as with any other project, must be carefully planned. But you must not lose sight of its effect on individuals. Depending on the nature of the change, you must also be sensitive to the effect it could (will almost certainly) have on your patients.

You first need to work out your strategy and agree a timeframe. You must have a start date and a finite implementation span, irrespective of whether or not the changes are to be introduced incrementally or all in one 'big bang'.

Set goals and milestones so that you can monitor the progress of the plan. This helps enormously with keeping the plan on schedule and within budget.

What are the changes going to mean for each employee? Are there going to be changes to people's status? Are their working habits going to be affected, for example, changes to their working hours, or will they be working with new colleagues? Will you be challenging their beliefs, for example by moving towards a more customer care-focused approach? Is their behaviour going to have to change because you are introducing new working practices?

Change is stressful if it is imposed, so you must give your employees the opportunity to voice their concerns and to offer feedback. There will be criticism, which you must listen to. Uncertainty breeds anxiety, so you must be honest with everyone, provide as much information as you are able to and do not allow rumours to circulate. Try to anticipate the amount of resistance you might face and how much stress the whole process is going to place on you and your employees.

Motivating your employees during times of change is crucial. They will need to feel valued and have their fears and concerns acknowledged. Accept that people are motivated by different rewards. Learn the basic principles of motivational theory by reading, for example, about Maslow's hierarchy of needs. You need to understand what motivates people and how you can build a climate of honesty, openness and trust. You should never believe that you can 'buy' people by simply offering them more money. Ask yourself, 'What motivates me?' then find out what each of your employees wants from their job. Don't assume that everyone wants what you want.

Change is very unsettling. One practice my wife and I were involved with when we were providing management consultancy services was a prime example of this. The owner seemed to come to work every Monday morning with a new idea about how his employees should work. He didn't bother to talk to his staff beforehand, nor did he have any idea about how unsettling it all was. Plans for change must always be fully worked through *before* implementation, not after.

Improving the practice is one form of change that you might undertake, but another change programme is moving an NHS practice towards being a private practice. Converting to a private practice carries significant risks if it is not very carefully managed. Companies that operate private capitation schemes generally offer some help: they will always tell you about the number of practices they have already guided through the process, and about how easy it was. You must be cynical about their claims. Your patients and your practice are unique, and no outsider is going to know either of them as well as you do. Any change programme brings with it some degree of resistance, and if you sense that your patients will not accept a move towards private dentistry, heed the warnings. This does not mean that privatisation cannot be achieved but do not get swept along by other people's enthusiasm, which after all is nothing more than a sales pitch. If you do decide to use one of these companies to help you change your practice, you must remain in total control of the change process.

It's going back a few years now, but the moral of this story is still valid. I was asked to help a practice that had tried and failed to convert from NHS to private. The owners had been persuaded that 'conversion' would be easy, but a year or so down the line their business was in a bad way. They wanted to know how to get their NHS patients back. The mistake they had made was that they had not fully thought through their change programme, nor had they correctly evaluated the effect all of this would have on their patients. Maybe they had also overestimated patient loyalty.

22

Succession planning: your exit strategy

The book began by launching you on your career as a practice owner, but in time you will have to give some thought to how you are going to retire and dispose of or pass on your life's work. Everyone's circumstances are different, but what follows should give you some idea of why it is necessary to plan for this well ahead of time, and how you might go about it.

There is a disclaimer at the start of this book, but I want to specifically point out that what follows does not constitute financial or legal advice. You should always seek professional advice from your accountant and solicitor before making any decisions.

The ideal scenario is that you retire (at whatever age you have chosen) having found a buyer for your practice: your patients continue to be cared for, your employees keep their jobs, and everything continues in much the same way as it did previously. Here, you will have used the expertise of your accountant to finalise your tax affairs and draw a line under the business at a date chosen by you. Your accountant, solicitor and a practice sales agent will have ensured that you got the best price for the business and that all the legal red tape was handled correctly.

How do you achieve this 'perfect' situation? The short answer is that it is all about planning.

- Decide when you want to retire and sell the practice: I would do this at least 5 years ahead of time.
- Speak to your accountant maybe 2 years before the event so that you know what is involved from a financial and tax-planning point of view.
- Speak to your solicitor maybe 18 months to a year before the event so that you are aware of the legal aspect and so you know how long it is likely to take to wind up your affairs.
- Speak to a practice sales agent about a year before the event to start the ball rolling.

Not everything in life is that straightforward: sometimes because of illness or, in the worst case, death, things have to be done with more urgency.

Let's look at the situation where you suffer from a long-term illness and have to eventually (reluctantly) give up work and sell the practice. In a single-handed practice situation, if the owner is away from work for any length of time, and if there is no replacement dentist to step in and look after the patients, the practice can soon become worthless. Even when there are associates to fill in for an absent principal, things can soon begin to slide. In both these situations a lack of income from the practice can soon put pressure on the owner's personal finances, adding to their already high stress levels.

Hold this thought: you must have insurance to protect your personal income and insurance to cover the running costs of the practice, which should include the cost of using a locum.

There is not much you can do except find another dentist as quickly as you possibly can to maintain the practice turnover. If you are ill you will have to delegate this responsibility to someone else, preferably your spouse or partner. Although you probably won't want to talk about this in advance, it is worth talking to them about what would you do if . . .?

The death of the practice owner is the other situation you should plan for. Yes, no one likes to talk about this, but the more you plan and put in place arrangements in the event, the easier it is going to be for those left behind.

- Your solicitor should help you draw up a will so that your personal and business assets are protected as far as possible from any inheritance tax.

- Your accountant should be kept up to date about your financial affairs and should have access to all the information they are likely to need.
- Your spouse or partner should be knowledgeable enough to know how to go about selling the practice.

Rather than retiring altogether and making a clean break of it, you might opt for a phased exit, gradually easing down and working fewer days over a period of time, before finally giving up. This situation needs an even longer lead-in time from a financial and legal point of view than simply calling it a day.

> I had to give up clinical practice through ill health. I had to sell up, lock, stock and barrel. Apart from disposing of the physical part of the practice, my other concern was making sure that my patients (dentistry *is* a very personal business) continued to be cared for.
>
> I was a practising dentist for 25 years, and believe me that 25 years flew by; it is never too early to start planning for the day when you hand the practice keys over to someone else and walk off into the golden glow of your retirement.

You might at some point, however, decide that you simply want to sell your practice and move on to pastures new long before retirement. Having read this book, you should be familiar with the selling process.

23

A final thought

Working in a practice that is disorganised, either because it is badly managed or, worse still, because it is not managed at all, is extremely hard on your nerves. It leaves you mentally and physically drained. Before I unlocked the secrets of practice management I used to go home on a Friday night absolutely exhausted. Once I took control of the practice, instead of it controlling me, life became much easier.

This is a short poem I wrote that sums up my life 'pre-management'.

Monday morning
The weekend's done
Off to work
No time for fun.
Friday night
My work is done
Off to home
Too tired for fun.

I hope that what you have learnt from this book helps to make your Monday to Friday fun, and that your weekends are not just the two days in between when you try to recharge your batteries ready to do battle again.

The secret to managing the Genghis Khan way is being in control. As a practice owner and/or manager you have to sometimes be gentle, while at other times you will have to be severe and firm. You have to manage your practice with an iron fist inside a velvet glove.

Index